Stimulus Properties of Drugs

Stimulus Properties of Drugs

EDITORS

TRAVIS THOMPSON
Departments of Psychiatry and Pharmacology
University of Minnesota
Minneapolis, Minnesota

ROY PICKENS
Departments of Psychiatry and Pharmacology
University of Minnesota
Minneapolis, Minnesota

APPLETON-CENTURY-CROFTS
EDUCATIONAL DIVISION/MEREDITH CORPORATION
New York

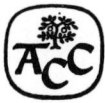

Copyright © 1971 by

MEREDITH CORPORATION

All rights reserved. This book, or parts thereof, must not be used or reproduced in any manner without written permission. For information address the publisher, Appleton-Century-Crofts, Educational Division, Meredith Corporation, 440 Park Avenue South, New York, New York 10016.

761-1

Library of Congress Catalog Card Number:
72-160809

RM
315
T 46

PRINTED IN THE UNITED STATES OF AMERICA

390-87603-8

DEDICATION

To the members of the Behavioral Pharmacology Society

Contributors

ROBERT L. BALSTER, Behavioral Pharmacology Section, Texas Research Institute, Houston Texas

GEORGE E. BIGELOW, Department of Psychiatry, University of Minnesota, Minneapolis, Minnesota

JOSEPH V. BRADY, Division of Behavioral Biology, The Johns Hopkins University, Baltimore, Maryland

A. CHARLES CATANIA, Department of Psychology, New York University, New York, New York

PETER B. DEWS, Department of Psychiatry, Harvard Medical School, Boston, Massachusetts

JOHN A. DOUGHERTY, Department of Psychiatry, University of Minnesota, Minneapolis, Minnesota

STEVEN R. GOLDBERG, Department of Pharmacology, Harvard Medical School, Boston, Massachusetts

ROBERT T. HARRIS, Behavioral Pharmacology Section, Texas Research Institute, Houston, Texas

HOWARD F. HUNT, Department of Psychiatry, Columbia University, New York, New York

KENNETH MacCORQUODALE, Department of Psychology, University of Minnesota, Minneapolis, Minnesota

J. BRUCE OVERMIER, Department of Psychology, University of Minnesota, Minneapolis, Minnesota

DONALD A. OVERTON, Eastern Pennsylvania Psychiatric Institute, Philadelphia, Pennsylvania

JORGE PEREZ-CRUET, Laboratory of Clinical Pharmacology, The National Heart Institute, National Institutes of Health, Bethesda, Maryland

ROY PICKENS, Departments of Psychiatry and Pharmacology, University of Minnesota, Minneapolis, Minnesota

CHARLES R. SCHUSTER, Department of Psychiatry, University of Chicago, Chicago, Illinois

TRAVIS THOMPSON, Departments of Psychiatry and Pharmacology, University of Minnesota, Minneapolis, Minnesota

MILTON A. TRAPOLD, Department of Psychology, University of Minnesota, Minneapolis, Minnesota

JAMES H. WOODS, Department of Pharmacology, University of Michigan, Ann Arbor, Michigan

Contents

CONTRIBUTORS		vii
PREFACE		xi
ACKNOWLEDGMENTS		xiii

	Section 1 INTRODUCTION	1
1	Interoceptive Stimulus Control of Behavior	
	Travis Thompson and Roy Pickens	3
	Section 2 UNCONDITIONED STIMULUS FUNCTIONS OF DRUGS	13
2	Drug Conditioning and Drug Effects on Cardiovascular Conditional Functions	
	Jorge Perez-Cruet	15
3	Conditioning of the Activity Effects of Drugs	
	Roy Pickens and John A. Dougherty	39
4	Nalorphine: Conditioning of Drug Effects on Operant Performance	
	Steven Robert Goldberg	51
5	Unconditioned Stimulus Functions of Drugs: Interpretations	
	I. Howard F. Hunt	73
	II. Milton A. Trapold	79
	Section 3 DISCRIMINATIVE STIMULUS FUNCTIONS OF DRUGS	85
6	Discriminative Control of Behavior by Drug States	
	Donald A. Overton	87

x   *Contents*

7	An Analysis of the Function of Drugs in the Stimulus Control of Operant Behavior	
	Robert T. Harris and Robert L. Balster	111
8	The Discriminative Control of a Food Reinforced Operant by Interoceptive Stimulation	
	Charles R. Schuster and Joseph V. Brady	133
9	Discriminative Stimulus Functions of Drugs: Interpretations	
	I. A. Charles Catania	149
	II. J. Bruce Overmier	157

	Section 4 REINFORCING STIMULUS FUNCTIONS OF DRUGS	161
10	Opiates as Reinforcing Stimuli	
	James H. Woods and Charles R. Schuster	163
11	Characteristics of Stimulant Drug Reinforcement	
	Roy Pickens and Travis Thompson	177
12	Environmental Variables Influencing Drug Self-Administration	
	Travis Thompson, George Bigelow, and Roy Pickens	193
13	Reinforcing Stimulus Functions of Drugs: Interpretations	
	I. Peter B. Dews	209
	II. Kenneth MacCorquodale	215

Index   219

Preface

Behavioral pharmacology represents a relatively recent scientific enterprise, the development of which can be followed by plotting the publication of major conceptual papers, review articles, and books. Dews (1955), Sidman (1955), and Brady (1956) published some of the first methodologically significant papers, changing the way both psychologists and pharmacologists viewed the analysis of the behavioral actions of drugs. Dews and Morse (1961), Cook and Kelleher (1963), Gollub and Brady (1965), and Weiss and Laties (1969) kept the field abreast of major developments in the study of behavioral mechanisms of drug action. In 1968, the first textbook in the field was published (Thompson and Schuster), followed by a book of readings covering the preceding 15 years of the field (Thompson, Pickens, and Meisch, 1970). The first attempt to outline a set of generalizations concerning behavioral mechanisms of drug actions was published in 1968 by Kelleher and Morse.

As behavioral pharmacology developed, it became clear that demonstrations that drugs affect behavior were relatively uninteresting. It was the *mechanisms* by which these effects are brought about that was of concern. While other aspects of pharmacology have been concerned with biochemical, physiological, and in some cases biophysical accounts of drug actions, behavioral pharmacology has dealt with behavioral mechanisms . . . that is, "any verifiable description of a drug's effects which can be shown to uniquely covary with a specific measured 'response'. Generally, this relation can be subsumed under some more general set of relations or principles" (Thompson, Pickens, and Meisch, 1970, p. 1).

Among the behavioral mechanisms by which drugs can affect behavior, one which has received considerable attention in recent years has been that drugs can serve as stimuli. Thus, much as visual and auditory stimuli can control behavior, drug-induced interoceptive stimulation can alter behavior as well. This book was an effort to bring together investigators working in the field, and to review their own and other findings concerning the possible stimulus functions drugs may serve. The major topics reported include eliciting, discriminative, and reinforcing functions of drugs. The findings have been exciting, revealing a new way of approaching the analysis of the highly complex interactions of drugs with environmental events to control behavior. Most revealing, in the words of one of the contributors to this volume, " . . . These results seem most remarkable to me for their congruence with the effects of other stimulus manipulations. . . . This orderliness and consistency pleases me, because it reassures me about the sensitivity and generality of our laboratory procedures, and the validity of our generalizations. . . . " (MacCorquodale, p. 217). This represents the importance of the work reported here. These data are part of a systematic approach to relate behavioral actions of drugs to principles and generalizations concerning behavior. It is this generality which makes them worthy of attention.

The editors are deeply indebted to the contributors to this volume, for their diligence and patience in arriving at a final publishable form of the book. Particular thanks goes to Gordon T. Heistad who was involved in the initial conception of the book, for his work in the early phases of organizing the book, contacting authors, and for his advice and guidance to the editors. The conceptual framework of the volume reflects our basic indebtedness to B.F. Skinner to whom our gratitude cannot be simply expressed. In addition, we want to thank Peter Dews, Roger Kelleher, William Morse, Charles R. Schuster, Lewis Gollub, Bernard Weiss, and Victor Laties for their contributions to our approach to behavioral pharmacology. We are grateful to them for all their work and writings which have shaped our thinking.

Brady, J.V. A comparative approach to the evaluation of drug effects upon affective behavior. Ann. N.Y. Acad. Sci., 1956, *64*, 632-643.

Cook, L. and Kelleher, R.T. Effects of drugs on behavior. Ann. Rev. Pharmacol., 1963, *3*, 205-222.

Dews, P.B. Studies on behavior. I. Differential sensitivity to pentobarbital of pecking performance in pigeons depending on the schedule of reward. J. Pharmacol. Exp. Ther., 1955, *113*, 393-401.

Dews, P.B. and Morse, W.H. Behavioral pharmacology. Ann. Rev. Pharmacol., 1961, *1*, 145-174.

Gollub, L.R. and Brady, J.V. Behavioral pharmacology. Ann. Rev. Pharmacol., 1965, *5*, 235-262.

Kelleher, R.T. and Morse, W.H. Determinants of the specificity of behavioral effects of drugs. *Ergebnisse der Physiologie*, 1968, *60*, 1-56.

Sidman, M. Technique for assessing the effects of drugs on timing behavior. *Science*, 1955, *122*, 925.

Thompson, T. and Schuster, C.R. *Behavioral Pharmacology*. Englewood Cliffs, N.J., Prentice-Hall, Inc. 1968.

Thompson, T., Pickens, R., and Meisch, R.A. *Readings in Behavioral Pharmacology*. New York, Appleton-Century-Crofts, 1970.

Weiss, B. and Laties, V.G. Behavioral pharmacology and toxicology. Ann. Rev. Pharmacol., 1969, *9*, 297-326.

Travis Thompson and Roy Pickens
Minneapolis, Minnesota
April 20, 1971

Acknowledgments

The present volume grew out of discussions over a number of years between Gordon T. Heistad and the editors. His early interest in interoceptive stimulus control of behavior played a significant role in gathering together many of the people most actively involved in the analysis of stimulus functions of drugs. Though he was involved in the planning and early editing, due to substantial commitments in the field of drug abuse education he was forced to withdraw from further participation in the book. Thus, while we have had the benefit of his ideas and suggestions, any errors and shortcomings in final composition and execution remain those of the editors.

Our deepest gratitude goes to the contributors to this volume whose work on stimulus properties of drugs form the fabric of the book. Having had the opportunity to assemble this collection of the most recent findings in this area of behavioral pharmacology has been most fruitful and enlightening to the editors. We are grateful to Jean Gaynor for manuscript preparation, and to Richard van Frank, of Appleton-Century-Crofts, for his patient cooperation in seeing this publication from conception through publication.

T.T.
R.P.

Stimulus Properties of Drugs

SECTION I
INTRODUCTION

Interoceptive Stimulus Control of Behavior[1]

Travis Thompson and Roy Pickens

Departments of Psychiatry and Pharmacology
University of Minnesota
Minneapolis, Minnesota

That behavior occurs differentially with respect to events occurring in the internal environment of organisms is well known. Investigations by neurophysiologists in the early 1800s left no doubt that afferent nerve fibers originating in blood vessels, the gastrointestinal tract, and the mesentery and urogenital systems carry sensory information to the brain. The receptors excited by stimuli arising within the organism were called *interoceptors*. By the middle of that century, pulmonary interoceptors controlling breathing, aortal receptors regulating cardiovascular responses, and deep muscle receptors concerned with coordinating reflex muscle activity were isolated and their functions studied. In 1880 Pavlov concluded that all internal tissues contained interoceptors capable of controlling unconditioned (reflex) responses (Bykov, 1957). It was not until almost 50 years later that interoceptors were found to be capable of controlling conditioned (learned) behavior as well.

RESPONDENT CONDITIONING

In respondent conditioning, a response comes to be elicited by a previously ineffective stimulus as the result of pairing that stimulus with one

---
[1] The preparation of this chapter was supported in part by USPHS Research Grants MH-15349 and MH-14112 to the University of Minnesota.

which normally elicits the response in question. The basic components of the respondent conditioning situation are

1. *Unconditioned stimulus* (US or UCS), a stimulus which evokes a regular and measurable response
2. *Unconditioned response* (UR or UCR), the response to the unconditioned stimulus
3. *Conditioned stimulus* (CS), a stimulus which initially does not evoke the unconditioned response
4. *Conditioned response* (CR), the response which occurs to the conditioned response as a result of CS-US pairings

In 1928, Bykov and Ivanova showed that an interoceptive stimulus could serve as the basis for the formation of a conditioned response (Bykov, 1957). They found that irrigation of the gastric mucosa in dogs would serve as a conditioned stimulus for a diuretic response. Subsequently, Bykov and co-workers explored an array of reflexively conditioned responses controlled by interoceptive stimulation. An aversive interoceptive reflex was established by pairing water irrigation of the stomach (CS) with faradic shock of the dog's hind paw. Discrimination of interoceptive CS was shown by pairing feeding with stomach irrigation of water at 36°C, while no feeding followed stomach irrigation of water at 26°C. Conditioned salivation came to occur only to the warmer of two conditioned stimuli (Bykov, 1957).

Investigations of interoceptive conditioned reflexes using drugs as unconditioned stimuli began with a report by Delov and Petrova (Bykov, 1957). They conditioned a cardiovascular reflex by pairing environmental conditions with the intravenous injection of large doses of morphine. Koniavi (Bykov, 1957) also demonstrated changes in blood pressure similar to those caused by the administration of morphine and hexanal alone, when a stimulus paired with the injection of morphine was presented. Collins and Tatum (1925) serendipitously discovered an interesting conditioned reflex during their study of the effects of daily injections of morphine on the dog. After seven or eight injections, their animals salivated not only after the injections but also before morphine was administered. The entrance of the experimenter into the room where the animals were kept was sufficient to elicit salivation, and at times emesis. This salivary conditioned reflex persisted as long as the daily injections were continued. Kleitman and Crisler (1927) replicated Collins and Tatum's experiment by systematically conditioning and extinguishing salivary conditioned reflexes in dogs, using morphine as the US. They discovered that the respondently conditioned reflex deteriorated as a result of deprivation, and that it recovered to full strength on feeding.

Korol, Sletten, and Brown (1966) respondently conditioned responses of paradoxical salivation and classical mydriasis, using equivalent doses of atropine sulfate and atropine methyl nitrate. Since atropine methyl nitrate does not readily enter the central nervous system, it was concluded that these conditioned responses were the result of peripheral anticholinergic drug action. In another report by Lang, Brown, Gershon, and Korol (1966), unrestrained dogs were conditioned with equivalent doses of atropine and Ditran which produced a paradoxical salivary response and a respondently conditioned response of mydriasis. Katzenelbogen, Loucks, and Gantt (1939) attempted to respondently condition salivation using adrenaline and histamine as the unconditioned stimuli. They failed to obtain conditioning of these reflexes, which was interpreted as indicating that the drugs acted only peripherally and had no central effects.

Pilocarpine, like morphine, injected subcutaneously in dogs evokes profuse salivation. Kleitman (1927) has reported that repeated injections of pilocarpine, unlike morphine, do not result in establishing conditioned salivary responses. This difference is apparently attributable to the fact that the two drugs act in different loci. Finch (1938) using dogs demonstrated that daily subcutaneous injections of 10 mg of pilocarpine hydrochloride resulted in a small progressive increase in preinjection salivary secretion. Withdrawal of pilocarpine resulted in a return of the secretory volume to the normal level.

Crisler (1930), in an effort to determine whether the actual elicitation of the unconditioned reflex was necessary for conditioning to take place, administered atropine to dogs prior to attempting to respondently condition salivation by the administration of morphine. Morphine induced a typical salivary conditioned reflex when the actual secretion of saliva was prevented by the atropine. Hence, the unconditioned response is not indispensable for the establishment of a typical salivary conditioned reflex.

Metalnikov and Chorine (1926) respondently conditioned leucocytosis, eosinophilia, and an increase in agglutination titer by presenting a loud bell or a thermal stimulus to the skin preceding injection of various antigenic or toxic agents into experimental animals. Smith and Salinger (1933) also demonstrated conditioned eosinophilia by respondently conditioning anaphylactic shock in guinea pigs. In addition to the eosinophilia, a variety of other motor responses such as coughing, labored breathing, scratching of the nose, voiding, and ruffling of the neck hair also became conditioned.

Herrnstein (1962) conditioned rats to press a lever for sweetened condensed milk reinforcement. Under specific stimulus conditions the rats occasionally received injections of 1 mg per kilogram of scopolamine, which suppressed responding. After repeated injections of scopolamine, injections of isotonic saline would produce a suppression of responding mimicking the scopolamine effect, apparently due to respondent conditioning. In a related study Levitt (1964) reported respondent conditioning of sleep. Rats were subcutaneously injected with various doses of morphine sulfate and degrees of activity and sleep were recorded. Though Levitt failed to obtain conditioned sleep in rats, however, when replicating the experiment with dogs, morphine and pentobarbital were found capable of inducing respondently conditioned sleep in that species.

Numerous investigators have attempted to respondently condition hypoglycemia or hyperglycemia. Gantt, Katzenelbogen, and Loucks (1937) attempted to condition hyperglycemia in dogs and rabbits using adrenaline as the unconditioned stimulus. Though their attempt failed, they observed other conditioned responses. Reiss (1958) repeatedly injected rats with insulin to produce hypoglycemic reactions, and then substituted saline for the insulin injection. The results demonstrated that a reaction not unlike that associated with the insulin injection could be produced. Kamfor (1958) sham-fed 16 patients with glucose solutions or saccharin, and observed rises in blood sugar for periods up to three hours after the sham-feeding. Administration of glucose directly into the stomach caused an increase in blood-sugar for one and one-half hours with a subsequent fall. Administration of saccharin directly into the stomach produces no change in blood sugar level. Balagura (1968) conditioned hyperglycemia in the rat using glucagon injections as the US and the injection procedure alone as the CS. A conditioned increase in an instrumental response for food was obtained using insulin as the US and the injection procedure as the CS. Woods, Makous, and Hutton (1968) demonstrated that rats who received insulin injections for fifteen days actually developed conditioned lowered blood glucose levels after a saline injection on the sixteenth day.

INTEROCEPTIVE STIMULUS CONTROL OF OPERANT BEHAVIOR

Stimulus control refers to the relation of an antecedent stimulus to the probability of an operant response. Interoceptive stimulus control of operant behavior largely went uninvestigated until recent years. Several early studies suggested that animals could be trained to respond differentially to food and water deprivation states without additional exteroceptive stimulation (Hull, 1933; Leeper, 1935; Kendler, 1945; Amsel, 1949). Slucki, Adam, and Porter (1965) presented the first demonstration of interoceptive stimulus control of operant behavior by mechanical stimulation. They conditioned monkeys to respond differentially to the rhythmic inflation and deflation of a balloon inserted in a small Thiry-Vella intestinal loop.

Another approach to the study of interoceptive control of operant behavior has been via drug administration. Some investigators have interpreted changes in responding to "dissociation," and others to novel internal stimulus effects. Regardless of the theoretical model investigators bring to the data, the fact remains that functional relations between values of antecedent drug manipulations and the probability of operant responding can be specified and are similar to the functions relating intensity of exteroceptive stimuli and the probability that a pigeon will peck a key. Such covariations have led to the generalization that drugs are capable of producing internal stimulus changes which can act as discriminative stimuli for operant behavior.

Conger (1951) demonstrated that rats could be trained to respond differentially in the T-maze for food reinforcement, based on the administration of ethanol or placebo. Stewart (1962) trained rats to respond differentially to the presence or absence of chlorpromazine. In a related study Heistad (1958) showed that conditioned suppression was differentially retained as a function of the presence or absence of chlorpromazine, depending on whether conditioning had been conducted in the presence of the drug or under placebo conditions. One of the better-controlled studies of interoceptive conditioning done in the United States was by Cook et al. (1959). These investigators demonstrated that conditioned avoidance responses could be brought under the control of the physiologic changes associated with the intravenous administration of epinephrine, norepinephrine, or acetylcholine. The administration of the drug solution acted as a discriminative stimulus for a leg flexion avoidance response by dogs.

REINFORCING FUNCTIONS OF DRUGS

"Of several responses made to the same situation, those which are accompanied or closely followed by satisfaction to the animal will ... be more firmly connected with the situation, so that, when it recurs, they will be more likely to recur ... " With the foregoing words, E.L. Thorndike first explicitly introduced the concept of reinforcement, and the notion that the future probability of behavior can be determined by the current consequences of responding. In efforts to objectively and operationally define reinforcement, Hull (1943) and Skinner (1938) provided experimental-procedural definitions of reinforcement. Whereas Hull's definition included theoretical terms such as "afferent receptor impulse," Skinner's approach was more purely operational. According to Skinner, a reinforcer is any consequence of an operant which increases the future probability of recurrence of the response which produced it.

The concept of reinforcement has proven important not only because it has provided the opportunity to bring an array of experimentally specified responses under control in the laboratory, but it has as well provided for an understanding of the acquisition and maintenance of a vast array of behaviors outside the laboratories. While most early investigations of reinforcement phenomena used food or water as maintaining consequences, investigations in the 1950s and subsequently have shown that a large number of "nonessential" substances or consequences can serve as reinforcers as well. Saccharin (Sheffield and Roby, 1950), the opportunity to look out a window from an experimental compartment (Butler, 1953), electrical stimulation of subcortical brain structures (Olds and Milner, 1954), heat (Weiss and Laties, 1961), and the opportunity to engage in aggressive behavior (Thompson, 1963, 1964) have all been shown to serve as maintaining consequences when made contingent on the occurrence of operant responses. Such reinforcers have been of interest since they have demonstrated that substances that do not reduce physiologic "need" can serve as effective reinforcers, and that consequences providing the opportunity to engage in other activities could also serve as reinforcers (Premack, 1959). However, whenever a new reinforcer is demonstrated to be effective in controlling behavior, the possibility remains that such reinforcers have properties different from previously demonstrated maintaining consequences. To determine the degree to which any newly discovered reinforcer differs from others, it is necessary to explore each of the variables known to control reinforcer efficacy.

Drugs as reinforcers. That drugs can serve as maintaining consequences for instrumental or operant responding is not a new notion. Spragg (1940) demonstrated that chimpanzees that were physically dependent on morphine would learn an instrumental response that would lead to the experimenter's administering the drug to the dependent animal. Subsequently, Beach (1957) showed a similar phenomenon with physically dependent rats. The first experimental demonstration that animals would actively administer drugs to themselves was by Headlee, Coppock, and Nichols (1955), who showed that rats would self-inject morphine, much as a hungry animal will learn to press a switch to receive food reinforcement. Subsequently, numerous investigators have shown similar phenomena in rats and monkeys using an array of drugs (Thompson and Pickens, 1969; Schuster and Thompson, 1969; Pickens, 1968).

SUMMARY

Thus, at least initial demonstrations have been made indicating that drug-produced states are capable of serving the same stimulus functions as exteroceptive stimuli, namely, unconditioned stimulus, discriminative stimulus, and reinforcing stimulus functions. One could agree with Skinner (1953) that such demonstrations primarily represent methodologic advances but minimal conceptual contributions if the only consequences of these observations had been the development of a technology. It appears, however, that explication of stimulus functions of drugs has both practical and conceptual implications that were difficult to anticipate. The clinically observed placebo effect, the disruption of behavior by the novel stimulus effects of drug states in nonpsychiatric as well as psychiatric patients, the widespread use of behaviorally active drugs which apparently serve as highly effective reinforcers (Schuster and Thompson, 1969), all illustrate the substantial practical implications of stimulus functions of drugs.

The conceptual implications are only beginning to emerge. While there is considerable evidence that the nature of the reinforcer is often less important than the maintaining contingencies (Morse and Kelleher, 1970), reinforcers are known to have different properties, not predictable from our knowledge of other reinforcers. For example, it appears difficult to maintain behavior by response-produced injections of hallucinogen drugs in animals, whereas humans frequently self-administer such agents. On continuous reinforcement schedules, the patterns of responding maintained by self-administered amphetamine or cocaine bear little resemblance to the pattern of food or water-reinforced responding. More importantly, our conception of the relation between magnitude of reinforcement and response rate based on short sessions of food and water reinforcement have been found to be erroneous, a discovery made using cocaine reinforcement. Subsequent investigations have revealed that such differences appear to be due to parametric features of typical food and water reinforcement studies, as opposed to drug-reinforcement experiments.

REFERENCES

Amsel, A. Selective association and the anticipatory goal response mechanism as explanatory concepts in learning theory. *J. Exp. Psychol.*, 1949, *59*, 785-799.

Balagura, S. Conditioned glycemic responses in the control of food intake. *J. Comp. Physiol. Psychol.*, 1968, *65*, 30-32.

Beach, H.D. Morphine addiction in rats. *Canad. J. Psychol.*, 1957, *11*, 104-112.
Butler, R.A. Discrimination learning by rhesus monkeys to visual exploration motivation. *J. Comp. Physiol. Psychol.*, 1953, *46*, 95-98.
Bykov, K.M. (translated by W.H. Gantt) *The Cerebral Cortex and the Internal Organs.* New York, Chemical Publishing Co., Inc. 1957.
Collins, K.H. and Tatum, A.L. A conditioned reflex established by chronic morphine poisoning. *Amer. J. Physiol.*, 1925, *74*, 14-15.
Conger, J.J. The effects of alcohol on conflict behavior in the albino rat. *Quart. J. Stud. Alcohol*, 1951, *12*, 1-29.
Cook, L., Davidson, A., Davis, D.L., and Kelleher, R.T. Epinephrine, norepinephrine, and acetylcholine as conditioned stimuli for avoidance behavior. *Science*, 1960, *131*, 990-991.
Crisler, G. Salivation is unnecessary for the establishment of the salivary conditioned reflex induced by morphine. *Amer. J. Physiol.*, 1930, *94*, 553-556.
Finch, G. Pilocarpine conditioning. *Amer. J. Physiol.*, 1938, *124*, 679-682.
Gantt, W., Katzenelbogen, S., and Loucks, R.B. An attempt to condition hyper-glycemia. *Bull. Hopkins Hosp.*, 1937, *60*, 400-411.
Headlee, C.P., Coppock, H.W., and Nichols, J.R. Apparatus and technique involved in a laboratory method of detecting the addictiveness of drugs. *J. Amer. Pharm. Ass.*, 1955, *44*, 229-231.
Heistad, G.T. Effects of chlorpromazine and electroconvulsive shock on a conditioned emotional response. *J. Comp. Physiol. Psychol.*, 1958, *51*, 209-212.
Herrnstein, R.J. Placebo effect in the rat. *Science*, 1962, *138*, 677-678.
Hull, C.L. Differential habituation to internal stimuli in the albino rat. *Journal of Comparative Psychology*, 1933, *16*, 255-273.
—— *Principles of Behavior.* New York, Appleton-Century-Crofts, 1943.
Kamfor, I.S. Characteristics of complex and reflex regulation of blood sugar level in man. *Bulletin of Experimental Biology and Medicine*, 1958, *46*, 899-901.
Katzenelbogen, S., Loucks, R.B., and Gantt, W. Horsley. An attempt to condition gastric secretion to histamine. *Amer. J. Physiol.*, 1939, *128*, 10-12.
Kendler, H.H. Drive interaction: I. Learning as a function of the simultaneous presence of the hunger and thirst drives. *J. Exp. Psychol.*, 1945, *35*, 96-109.
Kleitman, N. The influence of starvation on the rate of secretion of saliva elicited by pilocarpine and its bearing on conditioned salivation. *Amer. J. Physiol.*, 1927, *82*, 686-692.
—— and Crisler, G. A quantitative study of a salivary conditioned reflex. *Amer. J. Physiol.*, 1927, *79*, 571-614.
Korol, B., Sletten, I.W., and Brown, M.L. Conditioned physiological adaptation to anticholinergic drugs. *Amer. J. Physiol.*, 1966, *211*, 911-914.
Lang, W.J., Brown, M.L., Gershon, S., and Korol, B. Classical and physiological adaptive conditioned responses to anticholinergic drugs in conscious dogs. *Int. J. Neuropharmacol.*, 1966, *5*, 311-315.
Leeper, R. The role of motivation in learning: A. Study of the phenomenon of differential motivational control of the utilization of habits. *J. Genet. Psychol.*, 1935, *46*, 3-40.
Levitt, R.A. Sleep as a conditioned response. *Psychonomic Science*, 1964, *1*, 273-274.
Metalnikov, S. and Chorine, V. Rôle des réflexes conditionnels dans l'immunité. *Ann. Inst. Pasteur*, 1926, *40*, 893-900.
Morse, W.H. Intermittent reinforcement. *In* W.H. Honig, ed. *Operant Behavior: Areas of Research and Application.* New York, Appleton-Century-Crofts, 1966, 52-108.
—— and Kelleher, R.T. Schedules as fundamental determinants of behavior. *In* Schoenfeld, W.N. *Theories of Reinforcement Schedules.* New York, Appleton-Century-Crofts, 1970.

Olds, J. and Milner, P. Positive reinforcement produced by electrical stimulating of septal area and other regions of rat brain. *J. Comp. Physiol. Psychol.*, 1954, *47*, 419-427.

Pickens, R. Self-administration of stimulants by rats. *International Journal of the Addictions*, 1968, *3*, 215-221.

Premack, D. Toward empirical behavior laws. I: Positive reinforcement. *Psychol. Rev.*, 1959, *66*, 219-233.

Reiss, W.J. Conditioning of hyperinsulin type of behavior in the white rat. *J. Comp. Physiol. Psychol.*, 1958, *51*, 301-303.

Sheffield, F.D. and Roby, T.B. Reward value of a non-nutritive sweet taste. *J. Comp. Physiol. Psychol.*, 1950, *43*, 471-481.

Skinner, B.F. *The Behavior of Organisms: An Experimental Approach.* New York, Appleton-Century, 1938.

—— *Science and Human Behavior.* New York, The Macmillan Company, 1953.

Slucki, H., Adam, G., and Porter, R.W. Operant discrimination of an interoceptive stimulus in rhesus monkeys. *J. Exp. Anal. Behav.*, 1965, *8*, 405-414.

Smith, G.H. and Salinger, R. Hyper-sensitiveness and the conditioned reflex. *Yale J. Biol. Med.*, 1933, *5*, 387-402.

Spragg, S.D.S. Morphine addiction in chimpanzees. *Comparative Psychology Monograph*, 1940, *15*, #7.

Thompson, T. Visual reinforcement in Siamese fighting fish. *Science*, 1963, *141*, 55-56.

—— Visual reinforcement in fighting cocks. *J. Exp. Anal. Behav.*, 1964, 7, 45-49.

—— and Pickens, R. Drug self-administration and conditioning. *In* Hannah Steinberg, ed. *Scientific Basis of Drug Dependence.* London, J. & A. Churchill Ltd., 1969.

Weiss, B. and Laties, V.G. Behavioral thermo regulation. *Science*, 1961, *133*, 1338-1344.

Woods, S., Makous, W., and Hutton, A. A new technique for conditioned hypo-glycemia. *Psychonomic Science*, 1968, *10*, 389-390.

SECTION 2

UNCONDITIONED STIMULUS FUNCTIONS OF DRUGS

Drug Conditioning and Drug Effects on Cardiovascular Conditional Functions[1]

Jorge Perez-Cruet

Laboratory of Clinical Pharmacology
The National Heart Institute
Bethesda, Maryland

> It is true that the nervous system is earthy, whereas behavior seems to be evanescent, but the interesting things are evanescent, and one must deal with them as they pass. —B.F. Skinner (Evans, 1969, p. 17)

The modern application of some old and general laws of conditional behavior to physiologic and pharmacologic problems is a novel phenomenon in American science. The general laws of conditional behavior were first explored and postulated by Pavlov (1928) and Thorndike (1911) some fifty years ago. Pavlov established that the fundamental process of conditioning was psychic in nature and that it depended on two major variables: a *conditional stimulus* and a *reinforcement*. More recently, with the discovery of the stimulus properties of drugs, the area of conditioning and behavioral science acquired additional dimensions in terms of both experimental and clinical applications. The present report concerns the use of drugs and classical Pavlovian conditioning procedures in the study of cardiovascular function.

To mention the fact that drugs have behavioral or reinforcing effects often sets the classical pharmacologists thinking in terms of neurotic or psychotic clinical behaviors. By behavioral effects, however, we mean much more, including the psychologic, psychophysiologic, or neurologic control of basic behavioral functions. Processes that are behavioral are not necessarily organic or unconditional. They may also be conditional, resulting from the pairing of environmental stimuli. The experimental data we have accumu-

---

[1] This research was supported by NASA Grant NsG 520 and NIH Grant HE-06945 to The Johns Hopkins University School of Medicine, Baltimore, Maryland.

lated in this latter area over the past ten years may suggest possible applications for treatment and possible implications for the genesis of such pathologic states as essential hypertension and heart disease. Hopefully, therefore, we may be at the threshold of a new era in therapeutics, with the application of behavioral techniques for the treatment of disease.

MODIFICATION OF THE CARDIOVASCULAR SYSTEM

The problem of modifying the physiologic state of the cardiovascular system with drugs is very old. For example, the treatment of congestive heart failure with the leaves of common foxglove (digitalis) was discovered by trial and error many years ago. For centuries the effects of drugs on pathologic conditions of vital systems have dealt with the unconditional effects of drugs on such systems. We are only beginning to use drugs to examine the conditional modification of these systems.

The conditioning of drug effects on cardiovascular functions involves two general paradigms: (1) the actual conditioning of "specific" drug effects, namely, "specific" pharmacologic conditioning ("specific" in this sense is used here to state the nature of the response but not its mediation, origin, and complexity), and (2) the primary and secondary effects of drugs on cardiovascular conditioning. In the first paradigm a conditional stimulus (CS) usually precedes the injection of a drug known to produce specific unconditional effects, such as alterations in the electrocardiogram or changes in heart rate or blood pressure. After several repetitions of the CS and the drug reinforcement (unconditional stimulus or US), the CS is presented alone or followed by the injection of a neutral substance that does not produce pharmacologic effects. If conditioning has been established, the CS alone will produce changes similar or identical to the ones produced by the drug reinforcement. In the second paradigm, conditioning is established with a known agent such as cutaneous electrical stimulation to the skin or food, and the effects of drugs on this already established cardiac conditional reflex are determined. This method has been used in the past to determine the effects of certain tranquilizers on autonomic activity, but recently it has also been used to explore the physiologic mediation of these learned reflexes.

Early accounts of investigations concerning specific conditioning of the electrocardiogram were first reported by Bykov (1957). According to Bykov, the actions of morphine, nitroglycerin, strophanthin, epinephrine, and acetylcholine have been conditioned by various Russian investigators working in Pavlov's laboratories. The conditioning of the effects of morphine on the electrocardiogram was accomplished by Delov. After 30 repetitions of an injection of morphine paired with a complex CS, the complex CS alone came to produce conditional electrocardiographic changes similar to those produced by morphine, although morphine was omitted. Petrova studied cardiovascular conditioning using the sound of a whistle as a CS, reinforced with an intravenous injection of nitroglycerin. After about 30 repetitions of whistle and injection of nitroglycerin, Petrova obtained changes in the electrocardiogram to the whistle alone similar to those of nitroglycerin. A more distinct electrocardiogram conditional reflex to nitroglycerin was obtained after 100 reinforced trials. Conditional electrocardiograms have also been established by Samarin with strophanthin, and by Levitin with epinephrine and acetylcholine as the US. Teitelbaum, Gantt, and Stone (1956), on the other hand, were unable to condition changes in heart rate produced by acetylcholine. In 1956, Perez-Cruet in an unpublished thesis showed conditional changes in the electrocardiogram produced by two years of chronic emotional stress with classical defensive conditioning. Perez-Cruet and Gantt (1964) also were able to produce conditioning of the T-wave in the electrocardiogram with bulbocapnine as the US.

PHARMACOLOGIC ACTIONS OF BULBOCAPNINE

Our interest in conditioning the electrocardiogram with bulbocapnine arose from the fact that the chemical structure of bulbocapnine is very similar to apomorphine and morphine. The emetic action of apomorphine has been conditioned (Bykov, 1958) as well as the effects of morphine (Wikler and Pescor, 1966).

Figure 1 illustrates the chemical similarities between these alkaloids. Bulbocapnine is an alkaloid derived from corydalis cava, a bulb used since the Middle Ages for the treatment of convulsive disorders and tremors. The drug is not used intensively at present, although it was one of the first psychotropic agents introduced into neuropharmacology. DeJong (1945), in extensive studies with bulbocapnine, showed that this alkaloid could produce catatonic stupor in animals and man. According to some investigators the locus of action of bulbocapnine is in the diencephalon (Feldberg and Sherwood, 1955). Neurophysiologic studies with intracranial electrodes indicate the drug has inhibitory action in the Sylvian and cingulate gyri, amygdala, hippocampus, and reticular formation (Passouant, Passouant-Fontaine, and Cadilhac, 1955). At the enzymatic level, animals pretreated with bulbocapnine have a lower level of acetylcholine in the intracerebral substance than animals pretreated with LSD-25 (Poloni and Maffezzoni, 1952).

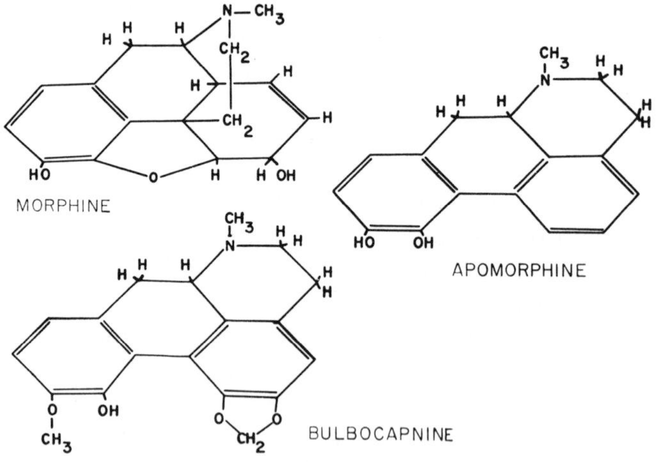

Fig. 1. Chemical structure of morphine, apomorphine, and bulbocapnine.

Figure 2 shows the electrocardiographic effects of bulbocapnine injected intracerebrally in the subthalamic region by means of a cannula described by Hernández-Peón et al. (1963). Injection of bulbocapnine only in this region produced a marked tachycardia and changes in the T-wave and bigemini. These changes began about 20 to 30 seconds after injection of 500 µg bulbocapnine and had almost disappeared 30 minutes later. These findings suggest the central action of the drug is in the subthalamic nuclei.

Experimental Procedure

In psychophysiologic experiments involving conditioning of autonomic behavior the animals are isolated from the experimenters to eliminate the effect of person, and the drug is usually injected from outside the experimental room. In this aspect our experiments differ from those of the Russian investigators in which the person was used as part of the complex CS. It has been shown that in some cases the effect of person on animals is as strong as the effects of some agents and physiologic maneuvers (Perez-Cruet, 1966b). The subjects used in our experiments were healthy adult mongrel dogs. The dogs were trained to stand on a platform inside a soundproof room, and they were observed through a one-way mirror. A total of 169 experimental sessions were performed over about 19 months. Standardized electrocardiograms, three standard limb leads and three bipolar chest leads, and a record

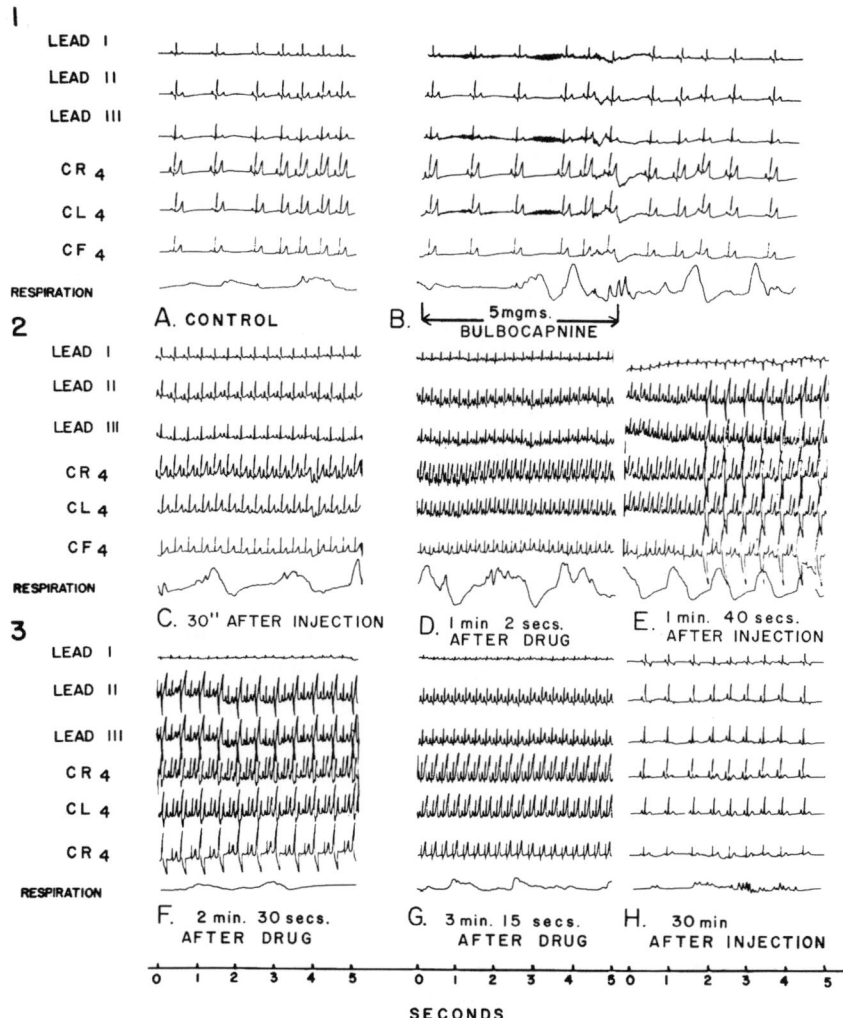

Fig. 2. Unconditioned EKG changes after intracerebral injection of bulbocapnine in the subthalamic region. 1A. Control tracings in standard leads 1, 2, and 3, and bipolar chest leads CR4, CL4, and CF4. 1B. Tracings during intracerebral injection of 0.5 mg of bulbocapnine. 2 C, D, and E. Various stages in the development of tachycardia, showing T-wave amplitude increase and extrasystoles after injection. 3 F and G. Bigemini, tall T-wave and accelerated heart rate shortly after injection. 3 H. Recovery without cardiac damage after 30 min. (Perez-Cruet and Gantt, 1964)

of respiration were taken concurrently with an Offner Type T recorder. A Fels cardiotachometer, Model 21-A, was also used to record instantaneous changes in heart rate. The injection of saline and bulbocapnine hydrochloride was through a fine polyethylene tube (P.E. 100, I.D. 0.034 by O.D. 0.060 inches) permanently implanted through the right external jugular vein into the right side of the heart.

Two previously neutral signals were used in conditioning: a low-intensity tone (500 cps) as the excitatory conditional signal (+CS), which was reinforced with bulbocapnine, and a flashing light (60 cycles/min) as the inhibitory conditional signal (−CS), which was never reinforced. The duration of these conditional signals was 15 seconds. The flashing light was always presented first and without injection; it was followed 2 minutes later by the tone, with the intravenous drug or saline injection occurring during the last 5 seconds of its presentation. The presentation of the tone plus drug injection corresponds to the reinforcement of the CS by food or faradic shock in the Pavlovian paradigm. One reinforcement was usually given each experimental day.

The criterion of electrocardiographic conditioning was based on the appearance of T-wave changes similar to those produced by bulbocapnine during presentation of the tone alone, provided the auditory signal had previously been reinforced with the injection of the drug ten or more times. Because of the fact that the cataleptic effect of bulbocapnine on motor behavior can last several hours, it was decided to determine the establishment of the conditional reflex in the electrocardiogram on experimental days in which no drug had been injected in the early part of the experimental session.

Controls

For each dog the effects of intravenous injections of normal saline and bulbocapnine, and presentation of the tone and flashing light on the electrocardiogram were determined prior to conditioning. The animals' normal electrocardiograms in both the sitting and standing positions were obtained.

The unconditional reaction to the flashing light and low-pitched tone, the orienting reflex, was also extinguished or obliterated prior to conditioning. The extinction of the orienting reflex was necessary because it has been found that this reflex produces significant changes in cardiac, respiratory, and motor reactions (Robinson and Gantt, 1947). The orienting reflex has been described by Pavlov as the general response of the subject to a new stimulus. It is characterized by turning of the head toward the stimulus.

Unconditional Cardiovascular Changes with Bulbocapnine

Figure 3 shows the electrocardiographic changes when bulbocapnine was injected into the right heart through an external jugular catheter. The drug produced marked tachycardia, tachypnea, and changes in the electrocardiogram consisting mainly of marked alterations in the amplitude and direction of T-waves. Frequently, inverted T-waves were reversed to an upright position, and, as a rule, upright ones were increased in amplitude. The changes in T-wave amplitude were more prominent for the bipolar chest leads than for the standard limb leads. The duration of the effect of bulbocapnine on the electrocardiogram was brief, an average of 2 minutes. If it were not for the fact that continuous records were taken, most of these changes would have been missed. In some experiments the electrocardiographic changes lasted 5 minutes or more, but seldom longer than 15 minutes. The intracardiac injection of bulbocapnine also produced marked tachycardia from 120 beats/min control to 240 beats/min peak response.

In other experiments, we have obtained similar results by injecting the drug through the cephalic vein in the foreleg instead of the external jugular vein.

Conditional Cardiovascular Changes

After 21 reinforced conditional trials, presentation of tone alone without injection elicited changes in the electrocardiogram similar to those produced originally by the drug. These results are shown in Figure 4. Heart-rate conditioning to bulbocapnine was usually established after two reinforcements whereas electrocardiographic conditioning required more. Heart-rate conditional reflexes were also more prominent than respiratory conditional reflexes (for heart rate: 104 beats/min during control and 204 beats/min during tone; for respiratory: 52 breaths/min during control and 60 breaths/min during tone), and the electrocardiographic changes were more labile than the heart-rate changes.

Figure 5 shows conditional heart-rate reactions after 30 reinforcements. There was complete differentiation in the autonomic functions with no heart-rate reaction to the inhibitory conditional flashing light (−CS), but marked tachycardia and tachypnea to the low-pitched tone (+CS). The

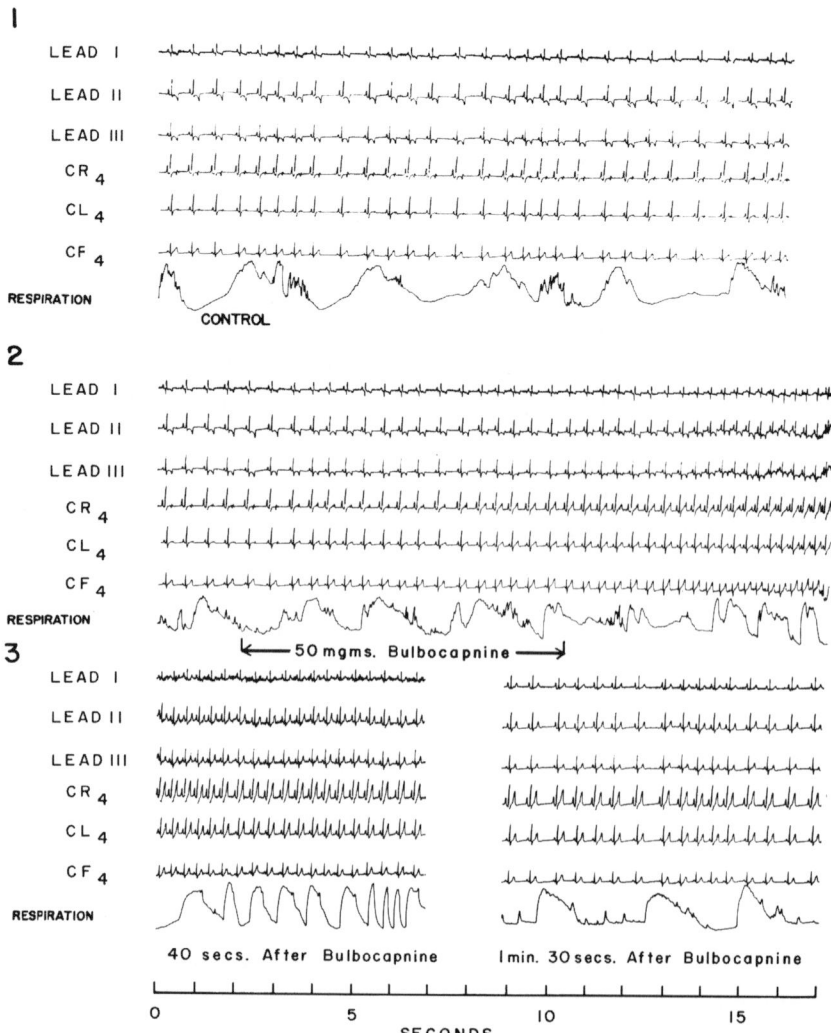

Fig. 3. EKG tracings showing the unconditioned effects of bulbocapnine injected into the heart. 1. Control EKG with sinus arrhythmia commonly seen in dogs. 2. Development of tachycardia 1 sec. after injection. 3. Unconditional tall T-waves in the presence of tachycardia and tachypnea (left tracing), and persistence of tall T-wave with regular sinus arrhythmia 1 min. 30 sec. after injection (right tracing). (Perez-Cruet and Gantt, 1964)

respiratory conditional changes usually preceded the beginning of the heart-rate conditional reflex. Differences were also seen in the relative speed of formation of respiratory, heart-rate, electrocardiographic and cataleptic conditional responses. In two animals, clear-cut conditioning of the catalepsy

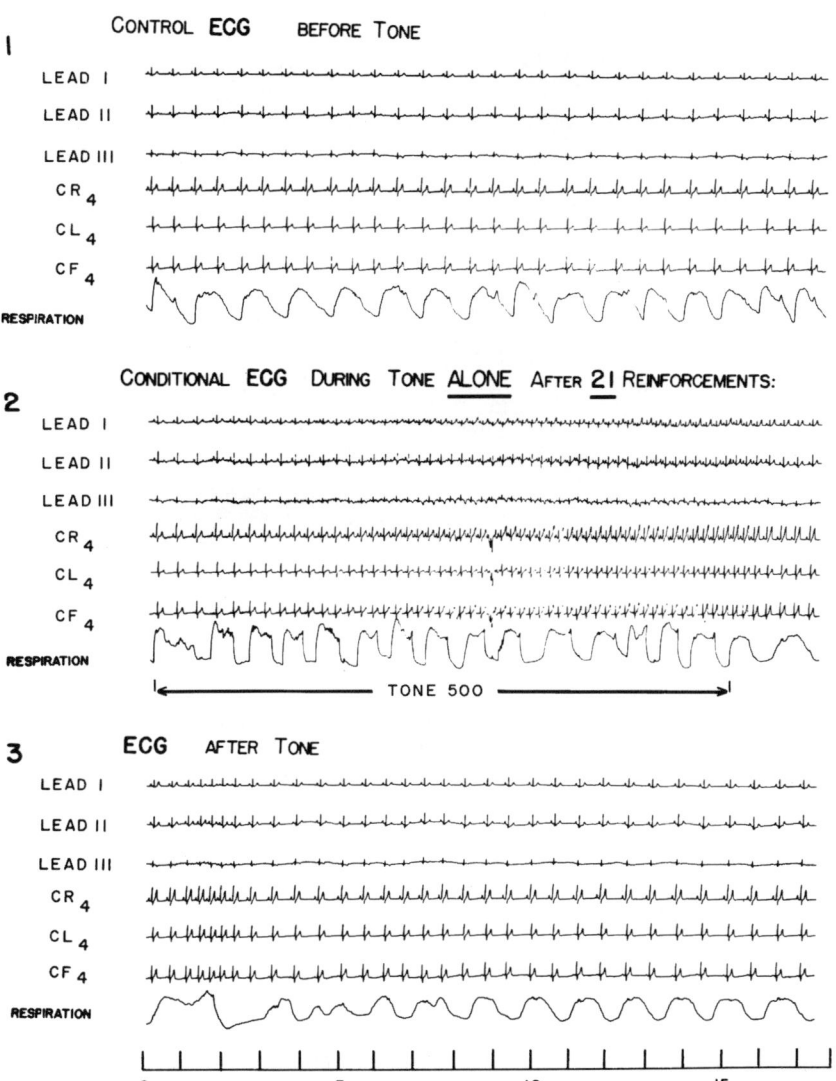

Fig. 4. Conditional EKG to tone alone after 21 bulbocapnine reinforcements. Tracings 1, 2, and 3 are continuous. 1. Control before tone. 2. Conditional EKG showing changes in the amplitude of the T-wave and tachycardia during presentation of tone alone. 3. EKG after tone showing persistence of a slight increase in the amplitude of the T-wave. (Perez-Cruet and Gantt, 1964)

produced by bulbocapnine was evidenced, and a third animal showed conditional immobility (Perez-Cruet, 1966a).

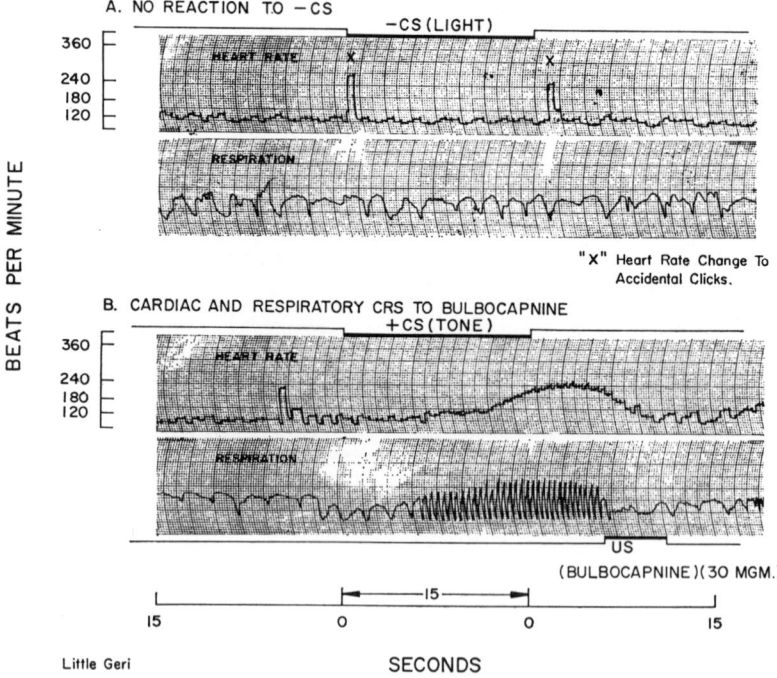

Fig. 5. Cardiorespiratory conditional reflexes to inhibitory (−CS) and excitatory (+CS) with bulbocapnine as the US. A. No reaction to the −CS. B. Heart rate and respiratory conditional reflex preceded the heart-rate CR. "X" indicates heart-rate changes produced artefactually. (Perez-Cruet, 1966a)

INVOLVEMENT OF CNS IN CONDITIONING

Previous work has shown that interoceptive conditional reflexes, based on stimuli arising within the organism, are as readily conditioned as somatic muscular responses. Pavlov (1910) began his conditional reflex work with autonomic responses such as gastric and salivary secretions. Bykov (1957) has conditioned vascular constriction and dilatation as well as cardiac reflexes. Burch (1961) has shown that the plethysmographic reflexes in humans can be conditioned as a component of the orienting reflex. Beier (1940) has conditioned blood pressure in humans and attempted to relate this to cardiovascular neurosis. Perez-Cruet (1962) conditioned extrasystoles in humans with respiratory maneuvers as the US.

It appears that at least one criterion for cardiovascular conditioning is

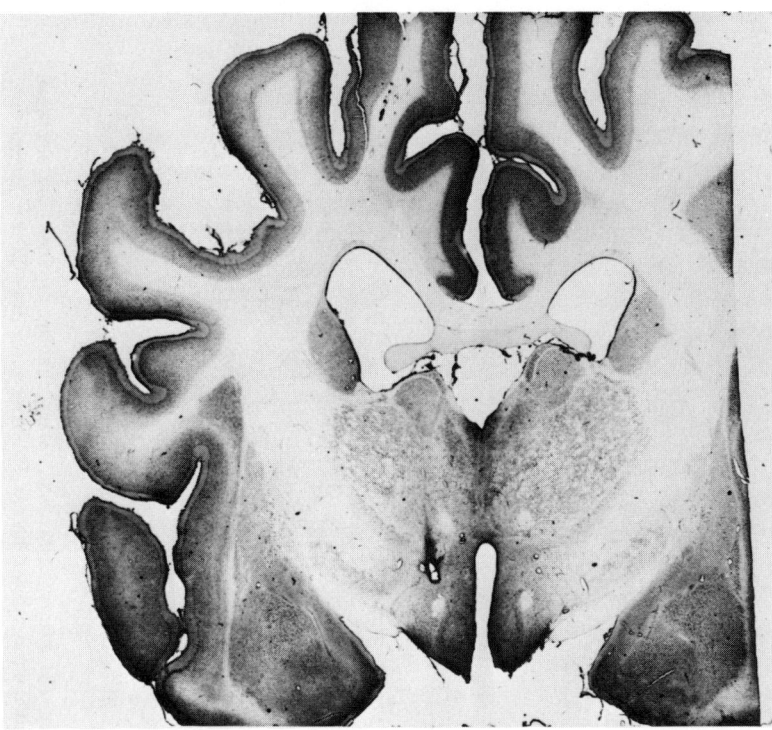

Fig. 6. Histologic section showing tip of electrode in the dorsomedial nucleus of the hypothalamus. Extrasystoles and T-wave changes were induced by stimulating this area electrically.

the involvement of the central nervous system in evoking the unconditional reaction. It is apparently the mechanisms by which the response is produced rather than the nature of the response itself that is important. Any response mediated by the central nervous system has a high probability of being conditioned. From our past experience, the effects of agents that produce their effects solely by peripheral action have not been amenable to conditioning. Peripherally elicited unconditional reactions such as tachycardia produced by atropine (MacKenzie and Gantt, 1950), gastric secretions produced by histamine (Katzenelbogen, Loucks, and Gantt, 1939), and hyperglycemia produced by adrenalin (Gantt, Katzenelbogen, and Loucks, 1937) have not been conditioned. When an agent produces some effects through the central nervous system and others via the periphery, it is believed that the central nervous system effects can be conditioned whereas the peripheral effects cannot. This is similar to "fractional conditioning" (Fleck and Gantt,

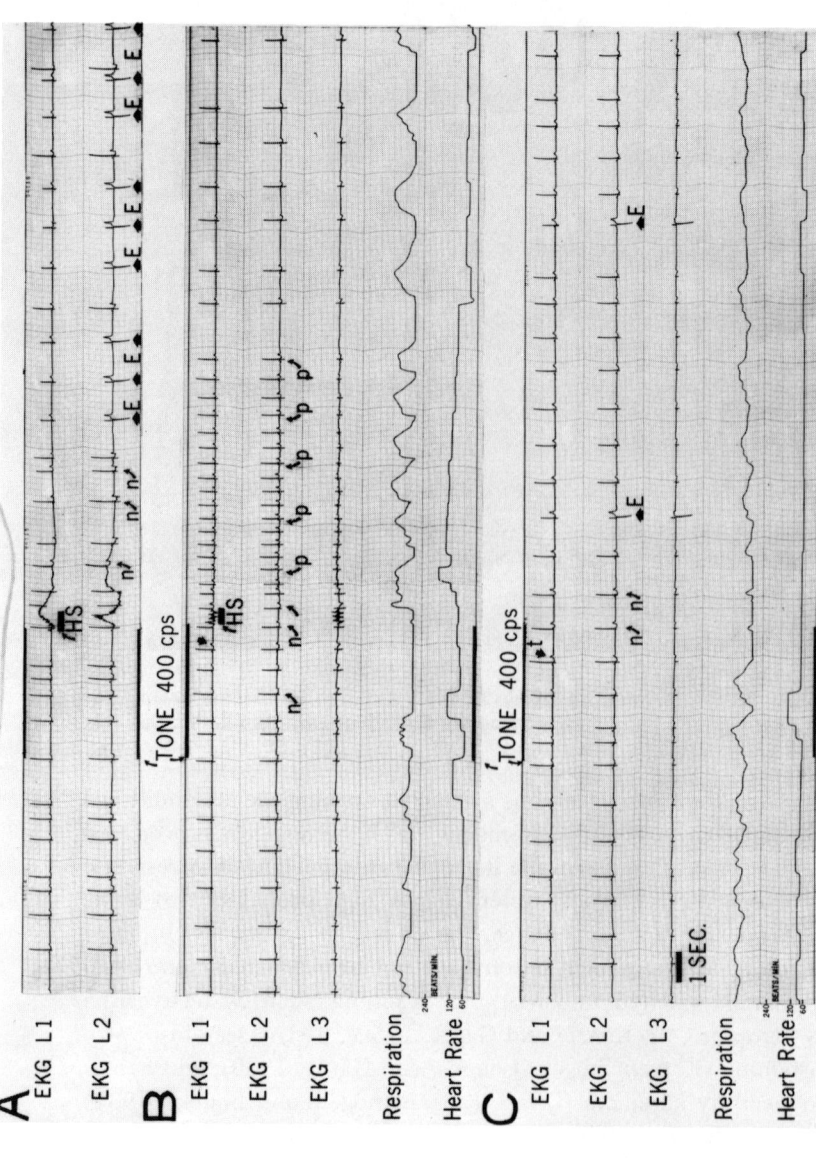

Fig. 7. A. Unconditional nodal (n) and ventricular (E) extrasystoles and T-wave changes produced by electrical hypothalamic stimulation (HS). B. Conditional nodal extrasystoles before HS after more than 20 reinforcements. Inversion of P-waves (p) and nodal tachycardia occurred in the EKG after HS. C. Conditional nodal and ventricular extrasystoles and T-wave changes to tone alone previously reinforced with HS more than 80 times. Note the cardiorespiratory conditional reflex in the respiration and heart-rate tracings.

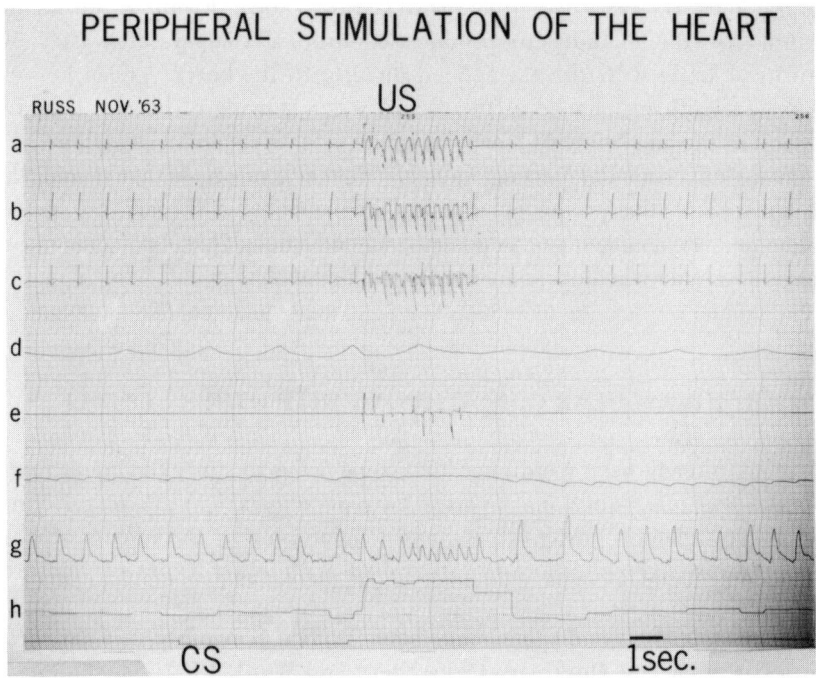

Fig. 8. Tracings showing no conditioning of peripheral extrasystoles after 594 reinforced trials, with US (electrical stimulation) applied directly to the myocardium. CS duration was 5 sec. Record lines a, b, and c are from EKG leads I, II, and III; d, respiration; e, US marker; f and g, DC and AC optical plethysmography (vasomotor activity); and h, heart rate from cardiotachometer. (Perez-Cruet et al., 1966)

1949). Perez-Cruet (1963b) has shown that some T-wave changes produced by intracranial stimulation of the hypothalamus are conditionable, but not easily so even when its origin is central. In these experiments, the location of the hypothalamic stimulation which produced T-wave changes and extrasystoles was in the dorsomedial nucleus of the hypothalamus (Fig. 6). These cardiovascular responses were elicited with a bipolar rectangular electrical stimulus of 100 cps and 1 ma for about 0.5 sec.

Figure 7 shows the conditional changes in T-wave and conditional extrasystoles produced by electrical hypothalamic stimulation. Not only electrocardiographic changes but also heart-rate changes have been conditioned with intracranial stimulation as the US (Malmo, 1965; Perez-Cruet, 1967, 1968).

It has also been shown that electrical stimuli applied directly to the heart muscle to produce extrasystoles, as a form of peripheral stimulation without nervous involvement, were not adequate for the establishment of conditional extrasystoles (Perez-Cruet, Jude, and Gantt, 1966). Figure 8 shows one example of the inability to produce conditional extrasystoles after 594 reinforced trials with the US applied directly to the heart. As can be seen, the only significant change in the record was a slowing of heart rate and an increase in the amplitude of plethysmogram after myocardial stimulation.

These experimental findings indicate a general principle that stimuli that act entirely at the periphery without involvement of the central nervous system are very hard, if not impossible, to condition. This also seems to be a general principle when drugs are employed as the US.

CARDIOVASCULAR CONDITIONING WITH OTHER STIMULI

It has already been mentioned that using drugs to study the conditioning of cardiovascular functions involves two paradigms: (1) the actual conditioning of "specific" drug effects, and (2) determining the effects of drugs on cardiovascular conditioning established with other types of reinforcement.

Cardiovascular conditioning has been studied previously in a variety of species (Cohen and Durkovic, 1966; Stern and Word, 1962; Schneiderman, Smith, Smith, and Gormezano, 1966; Anderson, Parmenter and Liddell, 1939; Smith and Stebbins, 1965; Perez-Cruet, Tolliver, Dunn, Marvin, and Brady, 1963). Newton and Perez-Cruet (1967) recently developed a successive-beat analysis for the study of cardiovascular conditioning. The usual method for evaluating changes in heart rate and blood pressure has been a comparison of averages of counts for five- to six-second periods before, during, and after CS presentation. This type of analysis gives no indication of beat-by-beat changes in cardiovascular parameters, which are important in the study of these reflexes. Our method for measuring heart rate and blood pressure resembles that used by Dykman and Gantt (1956) except that theirs involves a second-by-second analysis of heart-rate change. Zeaman, Deane, and Wegner (1954) used a similar method in studies of heart-rate conditioning in humans. The method of averaging successive heart beats before, during, and after a reinforced tone consists of aligning the first R-to-R heart wave intervals at the onset of the CS and summing them over several trials to obtain an average and standard deviation.

With this type of beat-by-beat heart-rate analysis, the cardiovascular conditional reflex to a tone reinforced by faradic shock has been found to be biphasic. An initial decrease in heart rate is followed by an increase. In dogs

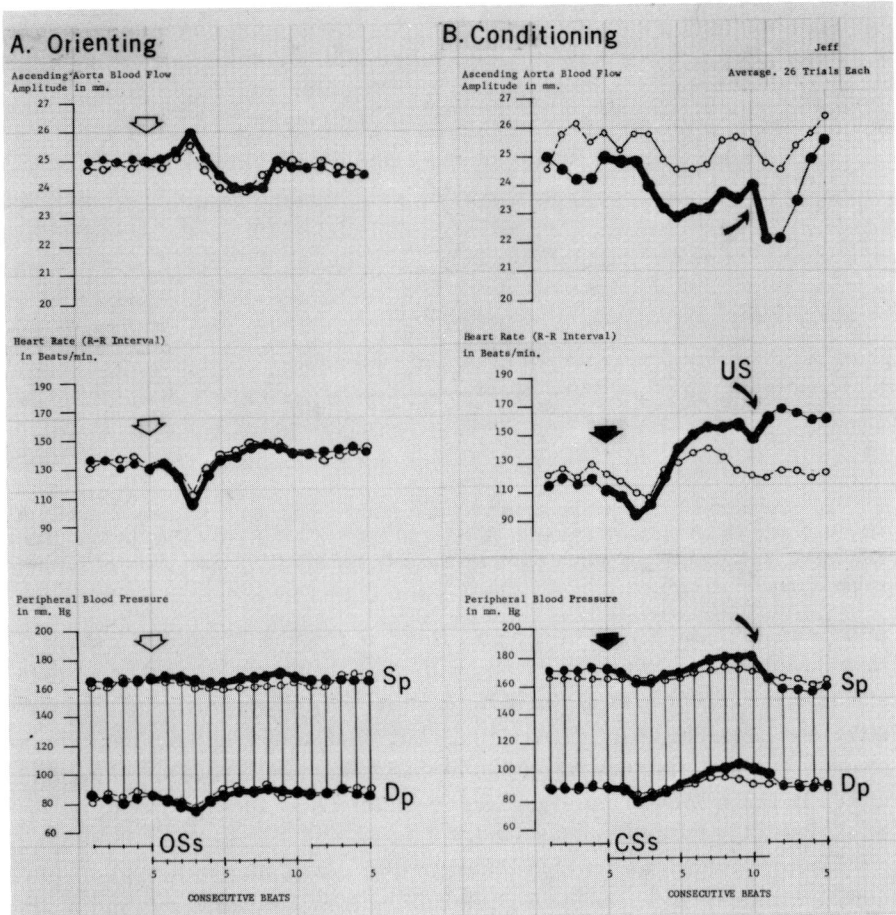

Fig. 9. Successive beat-by-beat analysis of cardiovascular conditional reflexes. A. Tracings of stroke volume (ascending aorta blood flow), heart rate, and abdominal aortic blood pressure during orienting. B. Tracings of similar measurements during conditioning. Curves with closed circles represent changes to +CS; curves with open circles represent changes to −CS. These tracings represent an average of 26 trials each.

these changes seem to be opposite to the initial acceleration followed by deceleration which has been reported for humans. The latent period for the heart-rate conditional reflex was 1.3 to 1.6 seconds or two to four cardiac cycles. Figure 9 illustrates a typical heart-rate conditional reflex with successive-beat analysis. As can be seen, the heart-rate change (middle tracing, column B) is biphasic, with the stroke volume decreasing and blood pressure increasing during conditional acceleration.

More recently not only heart rate and blood pressure, but a number of

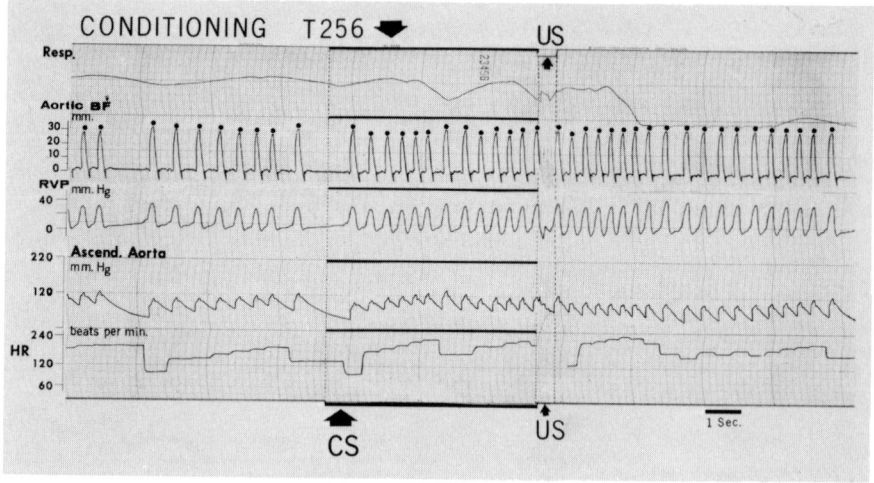

Fig. 10. Conditional changes in stroke volume (Aortic BF), right ventricular pressure (RVP), aortic blood pressure (Ascend. Aorta) and heart rate (HR) to a 256 cps tone (CS) reinforced with cutaneous stimulation to the left foreleg (US). See text for further explanation.

other variables, such as aortic blood flow, ventricular pressures, and caval flow have been measured chronically with implanted transducers (Perez-Cruet and Gaertner, 1966). It has been found that various cardiovascular parameters are physiologically interrelated, but that under certain conditions changes in heart rate can be either biphasic, acceleratory, or deceleratory, and that the hemodynamic variables seem to follow these heart-rate variations (Perez-Cruet and Gaertner 1968).

Figure 10 illustrates changes in respiration, ascending aortic blood flow (stroke volume), right ventricular pressure, aortic blood pressure, and heart rate during classical conditioning. As the tracings show, the US produced an increase in stroke volume, right ventricular pressure, and heart rate, but a decrease in systolic and diastolic aortic blood pressures. There was also a reduction in aortic blood flow during the early part of the heart-rate conditional reflex. This initial reduction in aortic blood flow is usually one of the earliest changes observed in cardiovascular conditioning. It is possible to speculate that the transient reduction in blood flow triggers some intrinsic cardiac reflex within the heart which allows for the physiologic mediation of the conditional heart-rate change.

Cardiovascular conditional reflexes are not obliterated by complete bilateral chronic cervical vagotomies in dogs, as shown in Figure 11. On the contrary, the reflexes become less variable due to the obliteration of sinus arrhythmia commonly seen in dogs (Perez-Cruet and Gaertner, 1967).

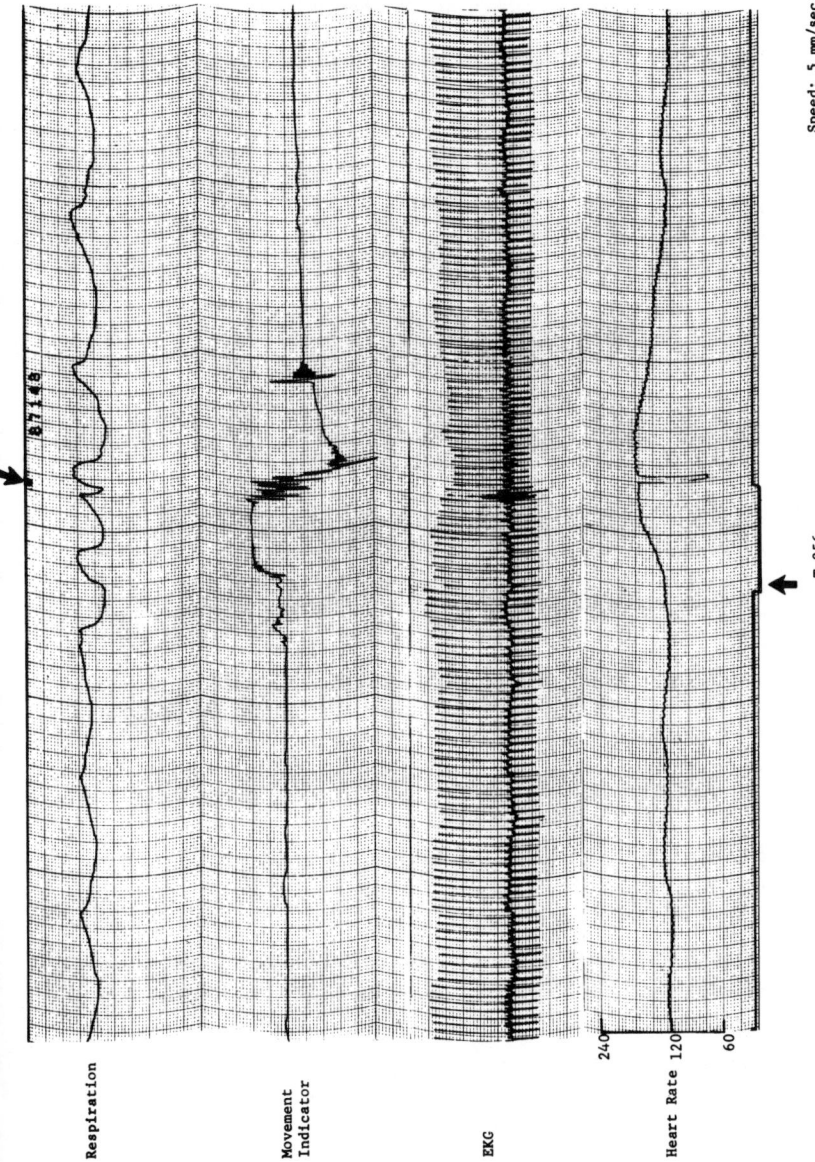

Fig. 11. Cardiorespiratory conditional changes in a chronically vagotomized dog during classical conditioning with cutaneous electrical stimulation as the US. Note conditional tachycardia and tachypnea during reinforced CS (T 256) presentation. A motor conditional reflex characterized by a foot-lift during the +CS is shown by the movement indicator.

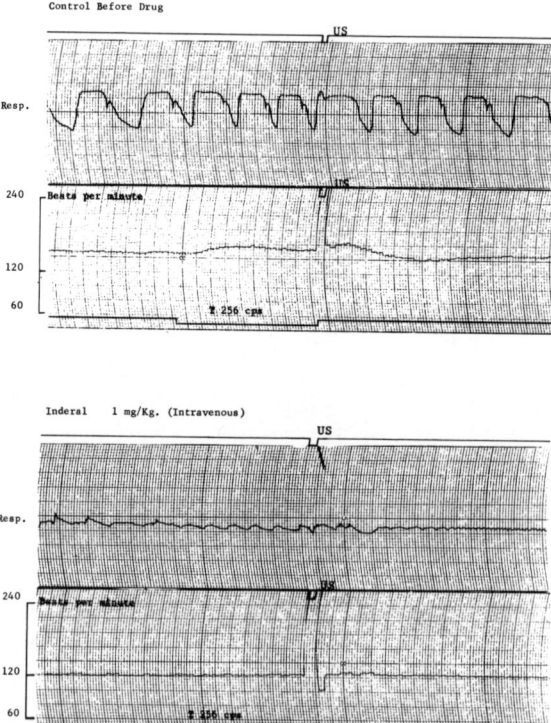

Fig. 12. A. Conditional cardiorespiratory responses in a vagotomized dog before injection of a beta-adrenergic blocking agent (propranolol). B. Complete blockade of the cardiac component, but no effect on the respiratory component after intravenous injection of propranolol (1 mg/kg).

DRUG EFFECTS ON CONDITIONAL CARDIOVASCULAR FUNCTIONS

If a vagotomized dog showing a well-established heart-rate conditional reflex is treated with the beta-adrenergic blocker propanolol hydrochloride (Inderal), the cardiovascular conditional and unconditional reflexes are completely blocked (Fig. 12). No effect, however, is seen on the respiratory conditional or unconditional reflexes. These results indicate that beta-adrenergic receptor mechanisms mediate the heart-rate conditional response in the vagotomized dog but that the respiratory conditional response is mediated by other mechanisms. In spite of the blockade of the cardiovascular reflexes by propranolol, there is no evidence of diminution in the

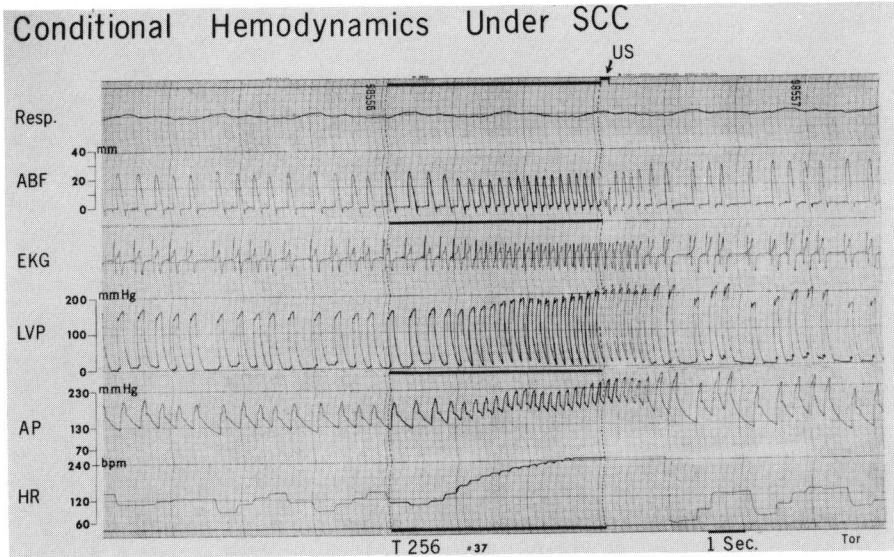

Fig. 13. Simultaneous tracings of respiration (Resp.), stroke volume (ABF), electrocardiogram (EKG), left ventricular pressure (LVP), abdominal aortic pressure (AP), and heart rate (HR) during complete musculoskeletal immobilization with succinylcholine (SCC), requiring that the animal be artificially respirated. These tracings illustrate that conditional cardiovascular changes can occur in a totally immobilized subject with controlled artificial respiration.

behavioral motoric reflexes consisting of a withdrawal of the reinforced foreleg during the CS presentation prior to faradic stimulation.

If an animal is treated with 1 mg/kg atropine, the baseline heart rate increases from an average of about 100 beats/min to about 240 beats/min. In spite of this shift in the heart-rate baseline level, the heart-rate conditional reflexes still remain, although not under atropine the magnitude of the response is diminished. If the atropinized subject is treated with propranolol, the baseline heart rate is reduced and the heart-rate conditional reflex is completely blocked (Perez-Cruet and Newton, 1967). It was evident from these studies that beta-adrenergic receptors and cholinergic mechanisms are involved in the mediation of these cardiovascular conditional reflexes. Studies in which the alpha-adrenergic receptors were blocked with Dibenzyline did not show clear blockade of the heart-rate conditional reflexes. Dibenzyline, however, seemed to have a more definite blocking action on blood pressure conditional reflexes.

In the past there have been controversies concerning the artefactual nature of visceral conditional responses. It has been stated by Smith (1954) that certain visceral responses may be due to artefacts of movements. Black

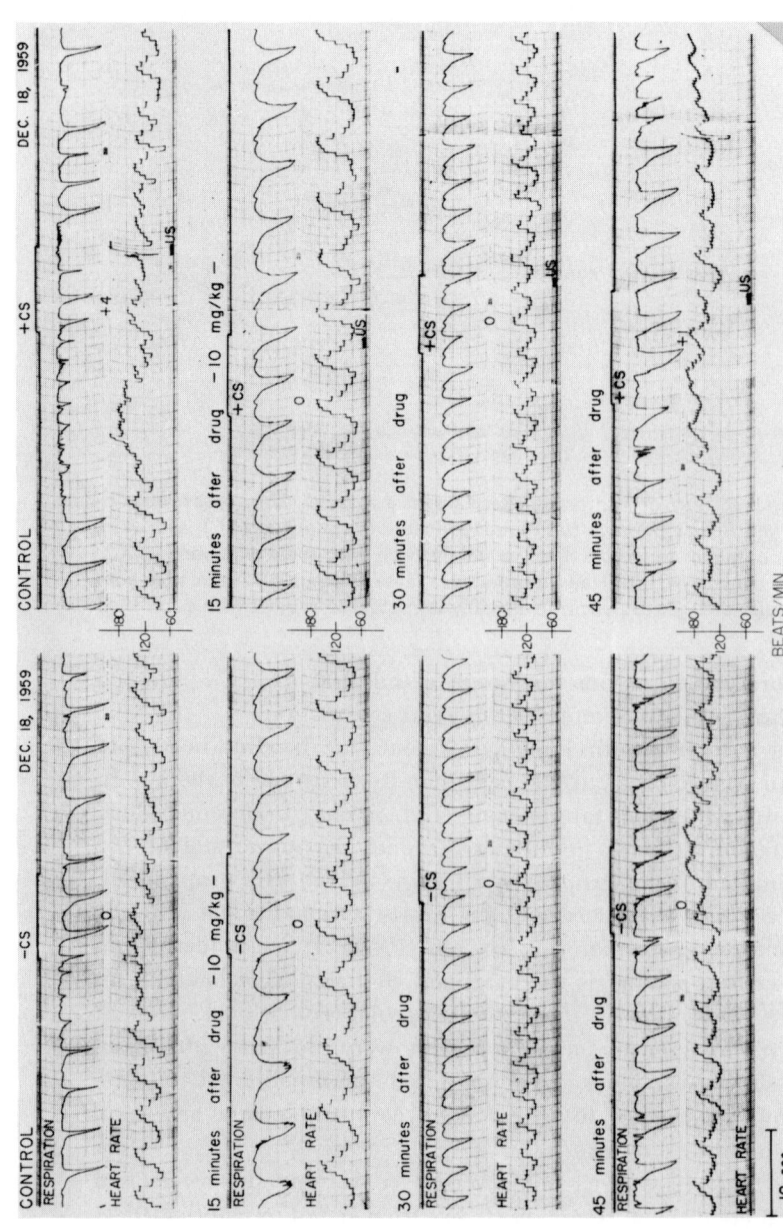

Fig. 14. Effects of acute bulbocapnine intoxication (10 mg/kg) on cardiorespiratory conditional reflexes. Control tracings show conditional reflexes to both inhibitory −CS and excitatory +CS, with cutaneous electrical stimulation as the US. Motor conditional responses are indicated as 0 for no response and +4 for a very strong response. Left column shows conditional changes to −CS and right column to +CS.

et al. (1962) were among the first to show that cardiovascular conditioning was not an artefact of movement and that it could be obtained in the curarized dog. Figure 13 illustrates various components of cardiovascular conditional reflexes in an animal paralyzed with succinylcholine (SCC) and ventilated artificially. A definite acceleratory heart-rate conditional response was observed under these conditions, with the left ventricular (LVP) and aortic blood pressure (AP) increasing and the stroke volume (ABF) decreasing. The experiments with curare and succinylcholine clearly show that these reflexes are not artefacts of musculoskeletal activity. At the same time, however, one has to consider that under physiologic conditions the muscular activity does play a major role in some of these responses, but it is not valid to state that they depend entirely on musculoskeletal feedback, as has been suggested by Obrist and Webb (1967).

Studies on the effects of drugs on cardiovascular conditioning are too numerous to review here. In general, the investigations in this field have shown that major tranquilizers, such as chlorpromazine (Thorazine) and reserpine, have a blocking action on heart-rate conditional reflexes (Gliedman and Gantt, 1956). Similar blocking action on cardiac conditioning has been found with mild sedatives such as meprobamate (Equanil or Miltown) (Gantt, 1964). Psychotropic drugs seem to have definite, but varied, effects on these reflexes. For example, mescaline, unless given in very high doses, does not block the heart-rate conditional reflexes (Bridger and Gantt, 1956). Bulbocapnine, on the other hand, has definite blocking action on cardiorespiratory conditional reflexes, as shown in Figure 14. In the figure, note that the anticipatory (time reflex) and conditioned cardiorespiratory conditional reflexes occurred to both −CS and +CS. Bulbocapnine intoxication produced catalepsy, and also blocked the cardiorespiratory conditional reflexes completely for 30 minutes, after which time they began to reappear, although catalepsy was still present (Perez-Cruet, 1963a).

SUMMARY

The study of cardiovascular conditioning is a useful tool for investigating visceral activity. It also permits a more comprehensive approach to the neuropharmacologic study of visceral function. Present studies indicate that there are many intricate interactions between external and internal environmental and pharmacologic variables controlling behavior. It is perhaps not too far from our reach to investigate these processes at the molecular and enzymatic level in order to find the fundamental biochemical and pharmacologic mechanism involved in cardiovascular conditioning.

REFERENCES

Anderson, O.D., Parmenter, R., and Liddell, H.S. Some cardiovascular manifestations of the experimental neurosis in sheep. *Psychosom. Med.*, 1939, *1*, 93.
Beier, D.C. Conditioned cardiovascular responses and suggestions for the treatment of cardiac neuroses. *J. Exp. Psychol.*, 1940, *26*, 311.
Black, A.H., Carlson, N.J., and Solomon, R.L. Exploratory studies of the conditioning of autonomic responses in curarized dogs. *Psychol. Monogr.*, 1962, *76*, (29, Whole No. 548).
Bridger, W.H. and Gantt, W.H. The effect of mescaline on differentiated conditional reflexes. *Amer. J. Psychiat.*, 1956, *113*, 352.
Burch, G.E. Digital rheoplethysmographic study of the orienting reflex in man. *Psychosom. Med.*, 1961, *23*, 403.
Bykov, K.M. *The Cerebral Cortex and the Internal Organs.* Trans. by W.H. Gantt. New York, Chemical Publishing Co., Inc., 1957.
────── *Textbook of Physiology.* Trans. by S. Belsky and D. Myshne. Moscow, Foreign Languages Publishing House, 1958.
Cohen, D.H. and Durkovic, R.G. Cardiac and respiratory conditioning, differentiation and extinction in the pigeon. *J. Exp. Anal. Behav.*, 1966, *9*, 681.
De Jong, H.H. *Experimental Catatonia.* Baltimore, The William & Wilkins Co., 1945.
────── A historical and personal approach to the development of experimental psychiatry. *J. Clin. Psychiat. Exp. Psychopath.*, 17:388, 1956.
Dykman, R.A. and Gantt, W.H. Relation of experimental tachycardia to amplitude of motor activity and intensity of the motivating stimulus. *Amer. J. Physiol.*, 1956, *185*, 495.
Evans, R.I. A dialogue with B.F. Skinner. *Psychiatry and Social Science Review*, 1969, *3* 11.
Feldberg, W. and Sherwood, S.L. Injections of bulbocapnine into the cerebral ventricles of cats. *Brit. J. Pharmacol.*, 1955, *10*, 371.
Fleck, S. and Gantt, W.H. Fractional conditioning of behavior based on electrically induced convulsions. *Fed. Proc.*, 1949, *8*, 47. (Abstract)
Gantt, W.H. Experimental studies in animals of the effects of drugs on cardiac stress symptoms. *J. Neuropsychiat.*, 1964, *5*, 472.
────── Katzenelbogen, S., and Loucks, R.B. An attempt to condition adrenaline hyperglycemia. *Bull. Hopkins Hosp.*, 1937, *60*, 400.
Gliedman, L.H. and Gantt, W.H. The effects of reserpine and chlorpromazine on orientiang behavior and retention of conditioned reflexes. *Southern Med. J.*, 1956, *49*, 880.
Hernández-Peón, R., Chávez-Ibarra, G., Morgane, P.J., and Timo-laria, C. Limbic cholinergic pathways involved in sleep and emotional behavior. *Exp. Neurol.*, 1963, *8*, 93.
Katzenelbogen, S., Loucks, R.B., and Gantt, W.H. Conditional reflex secretion. *Amer. J. Physiol.*, 1939, *128*, 10.
Malmo, R.B. Classical and instrumental conditioning with septal stimulation as reinforcement. *J. Comp. Physiol. Psychol.*, 1965, *60*, 1.
MacKenzie, T.M. and Gantt, W.H. Cardiac acceleration to atropine cannot be conditioned. *Fed. Proc.*, 1950, *9*, 83. (Abstract)
Newton, J.E.O. and Perez-Cruet, J. Successive-beat analysis of cardiovascular orienting and conditional responses. *Conditional Reflex*, 1967, *2*, 37.
Obrist, P. and Webb, R.A. Heart rate during conditioning in dogs: Relationship to somatic-motor activity. *Psychophysiology*, 1967, *4*, 7.

Passouant, P., Passouant-Fontaine, T.H., and Cadilhac, J. Modifications de l'excitabilité du cortex et de diverses structures sous-corticales au cours de la catalepsie provoquée par la bulbocapnine chez le Chat. *C. R. Soc. Biol.* (Paris), 1955, *149*, 2185.
Pavlov, I.P. *The Work of the Digestive Glands.* Trans. by W.H. Thompson. London, Griffin & Co., 1910.
—— *Lectures on conditioned reflexes.* Trans. by W.H. Gantt. New York, International Publishers Co., Inc. 1928.
Perez-Cruet, J. Conditional-reflex electrocardiogram in dogs. Thesis presented to the Award Committee, University of Puerto Rico School of Medicine, 1956.
—— Conditioning of extrasystoles in humans with respiratory maneuvers as unconditional stimulus. *Science*, 1962, *137*, 1060.
—— The effects of bulbocapnine on classical cardiorespiratory conditional reflexes. Paper presented at the Society for Psychophysiological Research, Detroit, 1963(a).
—— Electrocardiographic conditioning with hypothalamic stimulation as an unconditional stimulus. *Clinical Research*, 1963(b), *11*, 395. (Abstract)
—— Cardiorespiratory components of conditional catalepsy to bulbocapnine. In H. Brill ed. *Proceedings of the Fifth International Congress of Neuropsychopharmacology.* Amsterdam, Excerpta Medica Foundation, S. 129, 1966(a), 912.
—— The effect of person on heart rate in monkeys. *Clinical Research*, 1966(b), *14*, 257.
—— Chronic painless recording of intra-arterial blood pressure in unanesthetized dogs. *Conditioned Reflex*, 1967, *2*, 80.
—— Heart-rate conditioning with hypothalamic stimulation as an unconditional stimulus. *Proceedings of the International Union of Physiological Sciences*, 1968, *7*, 344.
—— and Gaertner, R.A. Cardiodynamics of cardiac conditioning. *Clinical Research*, 1966, *14*, 257. (Abstract)
—— and Gaertner, R.A. Cardiac conditioning in dogs with chronic bilateral cervicalvagotomies. *Fed. Proc.*, 1967, *26*, 328. (Abstract)
—— and Gaertner, R.A. Hemodynamic changes accompanying various patterns of classical cardiac conditional reflexes in dogs. *Clinical Research*, 1968, *16*, 243. (Abstract)
—— and Gantt, H.W. Conditional reflex electrocardiogram of bulbocapnine: Conditioning of the T-wave. *Amer. Heart J.*, 1964, *67*, 61.
—— and Newton, J.E.O. Effect of b-adrenergic blockage by propranolol on cardiovascular conditioning. *Clinical Research*, 1967, *15*, 218. (Abstract)
—— Jude, J.R., and Gantt, W.H. An attempt to condition extrasystoles using direct myocardial electrical stimulation as an unconditional stimulus. *Conditional Reflex*, 1966, *1*, 104.
—— Tolliver, G., Dunn, G., Marvin, S., and Brady, J.V. Concurrent measurement of heart rate and instrumental avoidance behavior in the rhesus monkey. *J. Exp. Anal. Behav.*, 1963, *6*, 61.
Poloni, A. and Maffezzoni, G. Le variazioni dell' attivitá colinergica del tussuto cerebrale per effetto della bulbocapnina, della mescalina e della dietilamide dell' acido lisergico. *Sist. Nerv.* (Milano), 1952, *4*, 578.
Robinson, J. and Gantt, W.H. The orienting reflex (questioning reaction): Cardiac, respiratory, salivary, and motor components. *Johns Hopkins Hospital Bulletin*, 1947, *80*, 231.
Schneiderman, N., Smith, M.C., Smith, A.C., and Gormezano, I. Heart rate classical conditioning in rabbits. *Psychonomic Science*, 1966, *6*, 241.
Smith, K. Conditioning as an artifact. *Psycholo. Rev.*, 1954, *61*, 217.
Smith, O.A. and Stebbins, W.C. Conditioned blood flow and heart rate in monkeys. *J. Comp. Physiol. Psychol.*, 1965, *59*, 432.

Stern, J.A. and Word, T.J. Heart rate changes during avoidance conditioning in the male albino rat. *J. Psychosom. Res.*, 1962, *6*, 167.

Teitelbaum, H.A., Gantt, W.H., and Stone, S. Cardiac conditional reflexes can be formed to pain but not to acetylcholine. *J. Nerv. Ment. Dis.*, 1956, *123*, 484.

Thorndike, E.L. *Animal Intelligence: Experimental studies.* New York, The Macmillan Company, 1911.

Wikler, A. and Pescor, F.T. Classical conditioning of a morphine-abstinence phenomenon, reinforcement of opioid-drinking behavior and "relapse" in morphine-addicted rats. In H. Brill ed. *Proceedings of the Fifth International Congress of Neuropsychopharmacology*, Amsterdam, Excerpta Medica Foundation, S. 129, 1966, 831.

Zeaman, D., Deane, G., and Wegner, N. Amplitude and latency characteristics of the conditioned heart response. *J. Psychol.*, 1954, *38*, 235.

3
Conditioning of the Activity Effects of Drugs[1]

Roy Pickens and John A. Dougherty

Departments of Psychiatry and Pharmacology
University of Minnesota
Minneapolis, Minnesota

A number of studies have reported conditioning of the activity effects of drugs. In these studies, the eliciting or unconditioned stimulus (US) was an injection of a drug which produced a change in activity, and the conditioned stimulus (CS) was a neutral event, such as placing the animal in an activity cage, which was paired with the drug injection. As a result of the CS-US pairing, the presentation of the CS alone was found capable of producing a change in activity similar to that elicited originally by the drug itself.

The present chapter reviews the studies that have been reported in this area, and describes the results of new investigations. In reviewing the existing studies, special attention is given to factors confounding the interpretation of their results. In no way should this be viewed as a criticism of the studies, however, but rather as a way of emphasizing the drug-behavior interactions found in this type of research. These interactions involve the type of activity recorder used, the control of indirect drug effects on activity, and the influence of apparatus habituation on the animal's activity. For the most part, these interactions are not seen in the typical studies of classical conditioning.

TYPE OF ACTIVITY-RECORDING CAGE

Acute drug administration. The first attempt to condition drug activity was by Irwin and Armstrong (1961). They reported conditioning of the

[1] Preparation of this chapter was supported in part by USPHS Research Grants No. MH-14112 and MH-15349 to the University of Minnesota.

activity increase produced by methamphetamine, and the activity decrease produced by perphenazine and chlorpromazine. In the first part of their study, conditioning of activity was attempted following a single drug injection. Three groups (N=32) of rats were given a subcutaneous injection of perphenazine (0.2 mg/kg), methamphetamine (2.0 mg/kg), or saline (US), and two hours later placed in activity wheels for a two-hour recording session (CS). As a test for conditioned activity, the animals were placed in the activity cages with saline substituted for the drug solution. These conditioning test sessions were run at approximately weekly intervals for nine weeks, and the activity of the groups that initially received drug injections was compared to that of the control group, which initially received only saline.

During the test sessions, conditioned activity was seen in both experimental groups. For the animals that had received a single injection of perphenazine, the first test injection of saline produced a substantial decrease in activity in comparison to that of the controls, indicating that conditioning had occurred. On the second test session, the activity decrease was somewhat reduced, and by the third test session was no longer apparent. This gradual loss of the conditioned response would be expected due to extinction. The activity level of the experimental animals was essentially the same as the controls on test sessions four through six. On the seventh session, however, the activity of the experimental group increased noticeably, and remained well above that of the controls for the remainder of the test sessions. This conditioned activity "rebound" effect has not been reported in other studies of classical conditioning, and is therefore difficult to explain.

For the animals initially receiving a single injection of methamphetamine, the first test injection of saline produced a considerable increase in activity over that of the controls. The magnitude of the activity increase was even greater on the second test session, and remained at about that level through the last test session. Apparently no extinction occurred, suggesting that the activity increase may not have been due solely to conditioning. Perhaps some other mechanism was also involved which maintained a high activity level once it had been increased initially by drug action.

Two possibilities for such a mechanism are suggested by the type of activity-recording device used. The activity wheel turns as the animal runs (positive feedback), but does not stop turning immediately when the animal stops running (negative feedback). Apparently this negative feedback is aversive, as animals tend to prolong their usual periods of activity while in such devices (Irwin, 1961), thus avoiding the aversive consequences which inactivity produces. Methamphetamine, by increasing the animal's activity in the wheel, presumably increases the number of activity periods and therefore the number of inactivity-avoidance sessions the animal receives, resulting in the more frequent negative reinforcement of running. It may also be that the positive feedback from running in the wheel is initially somewhat aversive, and consequently suppresses running. Methamphetamine, by making the animal run more, would simply accelerate the habituation to this feedback and thus augment future running in the wheel. Either alternative would explain Irwin and Armstrong's results, and we do not know whether their results are due to conditioning alone, a combination of one or both of the alternative explanations and conditioning, or to one or both of the alternative explanations alone.

It is interesting that both explanations can also be used to explain the increase in activity observed in the latter test sessions of the perphenazine conditioned-activity suppression study. In order to do so, we assume that some conditioning did in fact occur on the first test trial, and that the subsequent extinction of the response on the second and third test sessions produced enough of an increase in activity to differentially reinforce activity by inactivity avoidance or facilitated habituation, thus functioning effectively as methamphetamine.

Chronic drug administration. In the second part of their study, Irwin and Armstrong studied conditioning of activity following chronic drug administration. Rats were divided into six groups (N=10) and given daily injections of saline for 9 days, followed by one of three doses of perphenazine or chlorpromazine for 23 days, followed by saline again for 7 days. At approximately weekly intervals a two-hour session in activity wheels was given two hours after the subcutaneous drug or saline injection. Conditioning was determined by the change in activity which occurred to saline following the drug administration period.

Analysis of the data indicated a statistically significant decrease in activity to saline in four of the six animal groups. The conditioned activity effect was seen in the groups which had received the low and intermediate doses of each drug (0.1 and 0.2 mg/kg perphenazine; 1.1 and 2.2 mg/kg chlorpromazine). No decrease in activity to saline, however, was seen in the groups which had received the highest dose of each drug (0.4 mg/kg perphenazine; 4.4 mg/kg chlorpromazine). This indicated the activity decrease to saline seen with the lower doses of each drug could not have been the result of a toxic drug reaction. A subsequent replication of the study with a slightly longer drug injection period (26 days) and 3.0 mg/kg chlorpromazine was also unable to demonstrate a conditioned response.

The failure to find conditioning with relatively high doses of perphenazine and chlorpromazine was surprising, since these doses produced the greatest activity decreases, and therefore the greatest unconditioned responses. Usually the magnitude of the conditioned response increases with the magnitude of the unconditioned response (Hilgard and Marquis, 1940).

It is perhaps important to note that in subsequent attempts to replicate both parts of their study, Irwin and Armstrong found the results to be quite unpredictable, and failed in approximately two out of three cases. Variables such as age, sex, experience in the activity wheels, or activity levels did not relate to the development of the conditioned response.

SUITABLE CONTROL GROUPS

Ross and Schnitzer (1963) studied conditioning of drug activity using a stationary-type activity recorder, thus avoiding the confounding effects that cage movement can sometimes produce. They randomly assigned rats to three groups (N=10) and gave one week of daily conditioning trial. One group of subjects received intraperitoneal injections of 3.0 mg/kg d-amphetamine followed by a 45-minute session in a photocell-type activity cage, a second group received similar drug injections but was then returned to the home cages, and finally a third group received only sham injections (needle insert) followed by 45 minutes in the activity cage. Thus, the first group received the CS-US pairing, the second group received the US only, and the third group received the CS only.

One week after the last conditioning trial, all groups received a sham injection followed by a 45-minute session in the activity cage. The group receiving the CS-US pairing was found to be significantly more active than the group that had received the CS only. Whether the increased activity of the CS-US pairing group reflects conditioned activity, however, is impossible to determine, since the CS-only group did not receive the drug at any time, and therefore did not constitute an adequate control group. Conceivably, the greater activity of the CS-US group was due to some untoward drug effect, which the CS-only group, of course, would not show. This conjecture is consistent with their finding that the activity of the group that received the US only was also significantly higher than that of the CS-only group. In addition, the mean activity of the CS-US pairing group did not exceed that of the US-only group. The latter group, in fact, was somewhat more active than the CS-US pairing group! These findings taken together indicate the increased activity observed on the test day was due, not to conditioning, but to having received the drug in the past. Even had conditioning been shown, the results could also have been interpreted as some kind of interference with apparatus habituation, as the authors themselves point out.

APPARATUS HABITUATION

Rushton, Steinberg, and Tinson (1963) studied the effects of a single drug experience on subsequent reactions to the drug. Presumably their results would reflect drug conditioning. In their study, rats were divided into four groups (N=15) and given two 3-minute trials, three days apart, in a Y-shaped runway. Activity was measured by the number of times the animals entered the apparatus arms. The animals were injected subcutaneously with saline or a mixture of amphetamine sulfate (0.75 mg/kg) and amylobarbitone sodium (15 mg/kg) 35 minutes before each trial. One group of animals received the drug mixture on the first trial and saline on the second, and a second group received saline on the first trial and the drug mixture on the second. Two control groups were run which received either drug or saline on both trials. Conditioning would be reflected if the animal's activity on the second trial was influenced by the substance injected on the first.

The results indicated just such an effect. For the animals receiving the drug mixture on the first trial, the response to saline on the second trial was much greater than that of the animals that had received saline on both trials. Furthermore, for the animals receiving saline on the first trial, the response to the drug mixture on the second trial was much greater than that of the animals that had received the drug mixture on both trials. On first glance, these results apparently indicate a conditioned activity change not only to the amphetamine-barbiturate mixture, but to the saline as well.

Without considering the possibility of conditioning, Rushton, Steinberg, and Tinson attempted to explain their results on the also likely basis of habituation. If, when given on the first trial, the drug interferes with the animal's habituation to the activity apparatus, then the animal's subsequent response to saline would be expected to be much greater than had the animal been given only saline initially, which would have allowed some habituation to occur. If saline had been given first and the drug later, then the habituation to the apparatus which would have occurred under saline would subsequently reduce the animal's response to the drug, in comparison to that of animals that received the drug on both occasions and therefore were not allowed to habituate. Whether the results of the study reflect conditioning or simply the drug's effects on the habituation cannot be determined from these data.

DRUG-ACTIVITY CONDITIONING

In an attempt to control for such habituation effects, Pickens and Crowder (1967) first gave rats (N=8) six hours of habituation to a photocell activity apparatus, and then paired the animals on the basis of activity scores during the last 30-minute habituation session. The experimental member of each pair was injected intraperitoneally with 1.5 mg/kg d-amphetamine sulfate and placed in the activity apparatus for 30 minutes. The control member was injected with saline and placed in the apparatus for the same length of time. Approximately three to four hours after the activity session, the experimental animals were given saline injections and the control animals were given drug injections. Thus, all animals received habituation, the same amount of experience in the activity apparatus, and the same number of drug and saline injections. The only difference between each animal pair was that one received drug-placement pairings whereas the other did not, receiving instead the typical pseudo-conditioning control procedure.

Following six daily conditioning sessions, all animals were injected with saline and placed in the activity apparatus for 30 minutes. The activity of the animals in the experimental group to saline was significantly greater than that of the controls. Apparently these results do indicate conditioning of the activity effects of a drug, although a more general and somewhat different interpretation of all of these results can be offered, and will be discussed later.

FACTORS INFLUENCING DRUG-ACTIVITY CONDITIONING

Factors influencing the conditioning of a drug activity have also been studied. The only study in the area, however, has been that by Pickens and Crowder (1967) (also see Pickens, 1965). They investigated the effects of CS-US interval and extinction on conditioning of activity elicited by d-amphetamine injection in rats. The CS was the injection procedure and placement of the animal in a photocell-type activity apparatus. In an initial study, dose-response measures were obtained to select the drug dose that yielded the greatest activity increase, and time-response measures were obtained to select session length, so that CS presentation occurred before, after, and about simultaneously with maximum US effect. On the basis of this data, the drug dose selected was 1.5 mg/kg, and session length was 30 minutes.

For six days before the start of the experiment the subjects were habituated to the activity cage by being injected intraperitoneally with saline and placed in the apparatus for 60 minutes. Habituation was found to be complete by the fifth day.

Following habituation, the subjects were randomly divided into four groups (N=4) and given nine weeks of conditioning. During conditioning the weekly schedule consisted of six training days followed by one test day. One group of animals was injected intraperitoneally with 1.5 mg/kg d-amphetamine immediately before placement in the activity apparatus for 30 minutes, a second group received the drug injection 30 minutes before placement, and a third group received the drug immediately after removal from the cage. A fourth group served as a control, receiving saline immediately before placement and the drug three to four hours later. On test days all groups received saline immediately before placement in the apparatus.

The results showed that between the last three habituation sessions and the first three-day block of test sessions, the groups that received the drug immediately before placement and the drug 30 minutes before placement were significantly more active to saline than the group that received saline before placement. The greatest gain in activity from the last one-hour habituation to the first 30-minute test session was also by the groups that received drug before placement and drug 30 minutes before placement. These groups were more active on the first 30-minute test session than they had been on the last one-hour habituation session, with their activity increasing by 45 percent and 46 percent, respectively. During that same time, the activity of the saline before placement group decreased by 30 percent, as would be expected since the session length from habituation to testing had been reduced by about one half.

There was no significant difference between the groups receiving saline before placement and drug after removal from the apparatus. The activity of the drug after removal group between the last one-hour habituation session and the first 30-minute test session decreased by 41 percent, which was roughly similar to that observed for the saline before placement (control) group. Following the initial change in activity, which occurred during the first week of conditioning, no further change was evident throughout the remaining test sessions.

For seven successive days at the end of conditioning the animals were extinguished. The extinction days were similar to the test days, except that a drug injection was given three to four hours after the activity session, to maintain the animals at the daily drug level of conditioning.

Significant group differences were found in activity between the last three-day block of test sessions and the last three days of extinction. During extinction the activity of the drug before placement and drug 30 minutes before placement groups decreased, while that of the saline before placement group increased and the drug after removal group remained unchanged.

No further studies involving the conditioning of drug activity effects have been found. It is apparent that such conditioning can be successful, however, and that a number of factors influence this behavior.

NEW INVESTIGATIONS

In all the studies reported above, either subcutaneous or intraperitoneal drug injections were used. In a recent exploratory study, however, we have conditioned drug activity using an intravenous drug injection as the US. Our animals were equipped with a chronic jugular catheter system, which allowed the drug to be injected automatically without interfering with the animal's normal cage movements. The advantages of using such a drug-delivery system in studies of this sort are many. The first and most obvious is the increased control obtained over the onset of drug action. After parenteral injection, the time the drug becomes an effective US for activity is not easily determined. The onset of drug action is also relatively slow, and the peak drug effect does not occur until 20 to 40 minutes after the injection. Because of the relatively long absorption time, the duration of effect is longer and a relatively large drug dose must be used, thus increasing the possibility for drug accumulation, causing possibly confounding toxic effects. With intravenous injection, however, the onset of drug action is almost immediate and the peak effect occurs very rapidly. Much lower drug doses can therefore be used, and the effective duration of drug action is shorter. A second advantage of using an automatic intravenous drug-delivery system is that it eliminates the aversive stimuli that are produced by hypodermic injection. The possibility of getting a conditioned activity increase would seemingly be lessened by pairing the aversive injection procedure with the drug's effect. Another closely related advantage provided by the intravenous injection system is that it avoids experimenter-organism interactions, which may influence the conditioning results, and the variability of the animal's response to the drug as well. With such a system, the animal lives in the activity cage for the duration of the study, and is protected from environmental distractions. Thus, animal and treatment variability should both be reduced. Finally, the use of the automatic intravenous-injection system makes it possible for a more discrete and therefore better-defined CS to be used. Previously, the CS in conditioned drug activity studies has been described only vaguely as some aspect of the procedure of injecting and placing the animal in an activity cage. For purposes of experimental manipulation, it is therefore not possible to ascertain the nature, intensity, or duration of the CS presentation. Furthermore, if the activity cage is used as part of the CS, then it is impossible to manipulate the CS in any way without also changing the activity-recording baseline. These many advantages suggest that the automatic intravenous injection system offers an improved methodology for studying the conditioning of drug activity effects.

Method and procedure. In the study in which we used the intravenous drug injection system, our subjects were four male Holtzman albino rats approximately 150 days old. The apparatus was an animal chamber 10 by 10 by 9 inches high located within a large sound-shielding box. The animal chamber contained food and water supplies, a small stimulus light, and an activity-recording device. The activity recorder was an Alton Electronics Ultrasonic Motion Detector which was sensitive to disturbances caused by an animal moving through an ultra high-frequency sound field.

Initially, the animals were placed in the activity cage for at least 24 hours to allow habituation to the situation and to the illumination of the stimulus light. During this time the stimulus light was illuminated for 2-minute periods at hourly intervals.

Following habituation, the animals were surgically equipped with a chronic jugular catheter and fitted with the necessary auxiliary protection and support hardware. They were then returned to the activity cage, and the catheter was connected to an infusion pump. For the next several days, hourly infusions of 0.5 ml saline were administered. The duration of the infusion was always 25 seconds. At irregular times the stimulus light was illuminated, and the stimulus light presentations were also paired with the hourly saline infusions to determine the effects of this contingency on activity. The hourly pairings consisted of a 2-minute light presentation, with a 25-second saline infusion occurring 1 minute into the light presentation.

Following the completion of this control procedure, two of the subjects were used to condition the activity effects of methamphetamine infusion, while the remaining two subjects were used in a pseudo-conditioning control experiment. In the conditioning experiment, two daily CS-US pairings were given 3 hours apart for 5 days. The CS was illumination of the stimulus light for 2 minutes, and the US was a 25-second, 0.5 mg/kg methamphetamine hydrochloride infusion, occurring 1 minute into the stimulus light (CS) presentation. Hourly injections of saline were given to insure proper functioning of the catheter system. Activity was recorded continuously throughout the experiment on print-out counters and the stepper pen of cumulative recorders. In the pseudo-conditioning control experiment, the animals re-

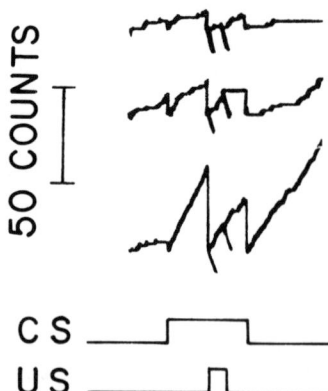

Fig. 1. Cumulative record segments showing development of conditioned drug activity. Each segment is five minutes in length.

ceived the same number of CS and US presentations as the animals in the conditioning experiment, except the CS presentation occurred 1 to 12 hours before the US presentation.

Results. Cumulative records showing the development of a conditioned activity response for one animal are presented in Figure 1. In the figure, pen resets designate different periods of activity for comparison. The top record segment shows the results of the final habituation trial before conditioning. As can be seen, CS-saline pairings have little influence on activity, with about the same number of counts occurring during the one-minute CS period before the onset of infusion as during the one-minute pre-CS (baseline) period. Saline infusion produced no noticeable activity change. The middle record segment shows the result of the third CS-US conditioning trial. The activity increase to the CS and US is readily apparent. The lower record shows the result of the seventh conditioning trial, where a marked increase in activity to the CS is seen.

In Figure 2, the data for the second animal are expressed in terms of the activity change occurring as a result of CS presentation. The activity count for the one-minute CS period prior to infusion was divided by that for the one-minute pre-CS (baseline) period to yield an activity change ratio. In the figure, the striped bar (0) represents the mean activity ratio of 72 CS-saline habituation sessions. The fact that this value (1.09) was essentially the same as the no-change value (1.00) indicates that the CS had little US activity effects of its own. The increase produced as a result of conditioning was much greater, being 3.02 and 3.44, respectively, for conditioning trials 1 to 5 and 6 to 10.

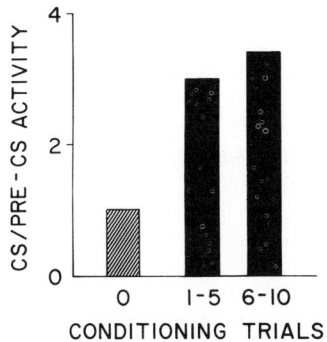

Fig. 2. CS/Pre-CS activity during saline control (striped bar) and conditioning (solid black bars).

In the pseudo-conditioning control experiment, the animals received the same number of CS and US presentations, except the CS-US presentations were non-contingent. No increase in activity was seen during CS presentations. This indicates that the results obtained in the conditioning experiment were not due to the drug's cumulative effects or lowering of the threshold for stimulation.

CLASSICAL OR OPERANT CONDITIONING?

While these findings therefore support the conditioning interpretation of the earlier results, there is one general criticism that can be directed against this and all other studies that purport to show the classical conditioning of the activity effects of drugs. The criticism is that the results obtained may be an operant phenomenon rather than classical conditioning per se. All of the drugs that have thus far been used in attempts to condition activity increases also serve as reinforcers of operant behavior. Since stimuli that signal the presentation of reinforcers come to generate increased activity (Sheffield and Campbell, 1954), it is possible the "classically conditioned drug activity" of the present experiments reflects nothing more than this effect. Studies of conditioned activity decreases do not offer support for either conditioning interpretation, as the reinforcing properties of the drugs used have not yet been determined for the rat. To separate the operant and classical conditioning effects, it would be necessary to demonstrate conditioned activity increases to drugs that do not also serve as reinforcers. Indeed, it would be interesting from a theoretical view to find such a drug, as the inextricability of these effects has been suggested by several learning theorists (Miller, 1963; Sheffield, 1954; Stein, 1964).

REFERENCES

Hilgard, E.R., and Marquis, D.G. *Conditioning and Learning*. New York, Appleton-Century-Crofts, 1940.

Irwin, S. The action of drugs on psychomotor activity. *Rev. Canad. Biol.*, 1961, *20*, 239.

—— and Armstrong, P.M. Conditioned locomotor response with drug as the unconditioned stimulus: Individual differences. In E. Rothlin, ed., *Neuropsychopharmacology*. Vol. 2. Amsterdam, Elsevier, 1961, 151-157.

Miller, N.E. Some reflections on the law of effect produce a new alternative to drive reduction. In *Nebraska Symposium on Motivation*. Lincoln, University of Nebraska Press, 1963.

Pickens, R.W. Conditioning of locomotor effects of *d*-amphetamine. Unpublished doctoral dissertation. University of Mississippi, 1965.

—— and Crowder, W.F. Effects of CS-US interval on conditioning of drug response, with assessment of speed of conditioning. *Psychopharmacologia*, 1967, *11*, 88.

Ross, S., and Schnitzer, S.B. Further support for a placebo effect in the rat. *Psychol. Rep.*, 1963, *13*, 461.

Rushton, R., Steinberg, H., and Tinson, C. Effects of a single experience on subsequent reactions to drugs. *Brit. J. Pharmacol.*, 1963, *20*, 99.

Sheffield, F.D. A drive induction theory of reinforcement. Paper read at Psychology Colloquium, Brown University, November, 1954.

—— and Campbell, B.A. The role of experience in the "spontaneous activity" of hungry rats. *J. Comp. Physiol. Psychol.*, 1954, *47*, 97.

Stein, L. Reciprocal action of reward and punishment mechanisms. In R.G. Heath ed. *The Role of Pleasure in Behavior*. New York, Harper & Row, Publishers, 1964.

4
Nalorphine: Conditioning of Drug Effects on Operant Performance[1]

Steven Robert Goldberg

Department of Pharmacology
Harvard Medical School
Boston, Massachusetts

When the morphine treatment of a physically dependent organism is abruptly discontinued, intense physiologic and behavioral signs and symptoms appear within a few hours of the last drug dose, reach a peak in intensity in 24 to 48 hours, and then gradually subside (Eddy, Halbach, Isbell, and Seevers, 1965; Jaffe, 1965). This complex of signs and symptoms, called the morphine-abstinence syndrome, includes anxiety, restlessness, disruption of ongoing behavior, increases in behavior motivated by drug acquisition, perspiration, salivation, mydriasis, body temperature changes, muscular aching and twitching, elevation of heart rate and respiratory rate, anorexia, and vomiting (Jaffe, 1965).

The abstinence syndrome may also be precipitated by administration of a specific morphine antagonist, such as nalorphine. In organisms physically dependent on morphine, the intravenous injection of nalorphine precipitates an abstinence syndrome within seconds that lasts for only a few hours (Jaffe, 1965; Woods, 1956). Minimal nalorphine doses, capable of precipitating an abstinence syndrome in organisms physically dependent on morphine, have no noticeable effect on nondependent organisms (Goldberg and Schuster, 1967, 1969; Goldberg, Woods, and Schuster, 1968). Except for time parameters, abstinence signs and symptoms precipitated by nalorphine and by abrupt termination of chronic morphine administration appear similar (Irwin and Seevers, 1952).

---

[1] Portions of this chapter are based on a dissertation submitted to the Graduate School of the University of Michigan in partial fulfillment of the requirements of the Ph.D. degree. This research was conducted with the aid of Dr. Charles R. Schuster and Dr. James H. Woods, and was supported by National Institutes of Health Training Grant 5R 10MH 12084.

The ease with which nalorphine precipitates the morphine-abstinence syndrome in physically dependent organisms has led to its frequent use by investigators as a tool to explore the behavioral and physiologic effects of morphine deprivation. For example, in the physically dependent rat, Weeks and Collins (1968) reported that continuous intravenous infusion of nalorphine produced dose-related increases in morphine self-administration and daily morphine intake. Similarly, Thompson and Schuster (1964) and Goldberg, Woods, and Schuster (1968, 1969) found that either morphine deprivation or administration of low nalorphine doses (0.1-0.3 mg/kg) increased morphine self-administration in physically dependent rhesus monkeys. Further, Goldberg, Woods, and Schuster (1968) reported that after testing these low doses of nalorphine, saline injections often increased the rate of morphine self-administration. Apparently, repeated association of the injection procedure with the abstinence changes elicited by nalorphine resulted in the injection procedure coming to produce conditioned changes in morphine self-administration.

The first experimental observation of a conditioned abstinence-like response to saline injection was made by Irwin and Seevers in 1956. Rhesus monkeys, physically dependent on the narcotic drugs, ketobemidone, racemorphan, and methadone, experienced repeated nalorphine-induced abstinence episodes. After one to two months without these drugs, about 25 percent of the monkeys continued to show an abstinence-like response to nalorphine, including increased salivation, vomiting, restlessness, lying down, and body tremors. When present, the "abstinence-like" response to nalorphine could be elicited by saline injection, extinguished by repeated injections of saline, and then reinstated by nalorphine administration.

These observations indicate that the effects of nalorphine injections may be classically conditioned to injections of more neutral substances. In Pavlovian terms, the nalorphine injection can be viewed as an unconditioned stimulus (US) and nalorphine's effects on morphine-dependent monkeys (abstinence syndrome) as an unconditioned response (UR). This chapter will review a series of experiments conducted at the University of Michigan which examined the acquisition, strength, and persistence of the conditioned behavioral and physiologic changes associated with the nalorphine-induced abstinence syndrome.

EXPERIMENTAL STUDIES

In many classical conditioning studies the rate of acquisition of the conditioned response is not measured, since the optimal interval (i.e., the interval producing the fastest rate of conditioning) between the onset of the conditioned stimulus (CS) and the onset of the US (CS-US interval) is often shorter than the latency of the conditioned response. As a consequence, when an optimal CS-US interval is used, the degree of conditioning can only be measured on occasions when the US is omitted. In addition to giving only fragmentary results, such a procedure introduces periodic extinction which can complicate and change the course of conditioning (Razran, 1956; Reynolds, 1958). This problem can be overcome by employing a CS-US interval sufficiently long to allow observation of the conditioned response in the interval between CS onset and presentation of the US. With the conditioned emotional response paradigm (CER), originally formulated by Estes and Skinner (1941), it is possible to follow acquisition in this manner. In this paradigm, a stimulus period (CS), which ends with an unavoidable electric shock (US), is superimposed on an intermittent schedule of food reinforcement, and the degree of food-responding suppression in the presence of the CS is then measured. Since this procedure allows simultaneous measurement of physiologic and operant behavioral changes, it was modified for use in a series of experiments by Goldberg and Schuster (1966, 1967, 1970) and Goldberg, Woods, and Schuster (1969), with morphine-dependent rhesus monkeys, by substituting nalorphine injection for the electric shock. Rather than terminating the CS with the onset of nalorphine injection, the CS continued for a period of time to insure overlap with the maximal unconditioned effects of the drug.

CONDITIONED CHANGES IN MORPHINE SELF-ADMINISTRATION

Method and Results. Details of this experiment have been previously reported (Goldberg, Woods, and Schuster, 1969). Briefly, three monkeys *(Macaca mulatta)* were surgically prepared with chronic jugular catheters and fitted with metal harnesses for restraint. Each monkey was housed in an individual cubicle equipped with a jointed metal restraining arm which was attached to the monkey's harness. The external portion of the intravenous catheter was contained within the restraining arm and led from the back of the arm to an automatic injector located behind the back wall of the cubicle. Each cubicle contained a lever, and each lever press at all times delivered an intravenous injection of 1.0 mg/kg morphine sulfate. Empirical details of experimental self-administration techniques for rhesus monkeys have been reported by Deneau, Yanagita, and Seevers (1969) and Yanagita, Deneau, and Seevers (1965).

Once drug self-administration responding was initiated, the morphine

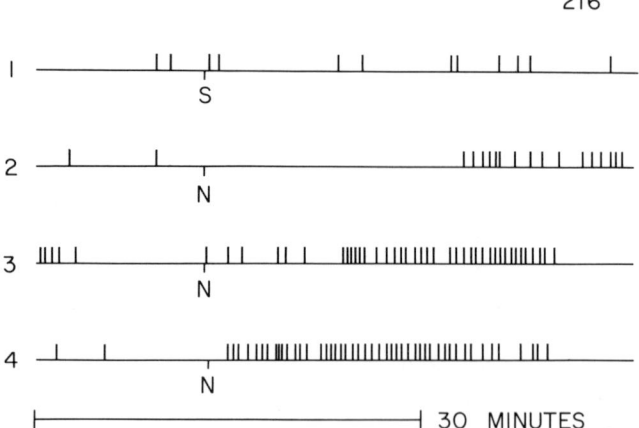

Fig. 1. Event records of Monkey 216 showing unconditional effects of saline (S) and 0.1 mg/kg nalorphine (N) on frequency of morphine self-administration for Day 1 to 4. Each injection is indicated by upward deflection of event pen. No light or tone CS was presented. (From Goldberg, Woods, and Schuster 1969. Science, 166:1306-1307. Copyright 1969 by the American Association for the Advancement of Science.)

dosage was gradually lowered to 0.1 mg/kg per injection. Monkeys were allowed access to morphine 24 hours per day, which resulted in a low response rate (an average of six responses per hour). When responding on this regimen stabilized (usually within 1 to 2 months, with 110 to 180 self-administrations or 11 to 18 mg/kg of morphine per day), a high degree of physical dependence on morphine could be assumed (Deneau and Seevers, 1964; Schuster and Thompson, 1969).

After stabilization of morphine self-administration, nalorphine (0.1 mg/kg) was administered intravenously on successive days to determine its unconditioned effects on responding. The results of these daily nalorphine injections are shown in Figure 1 for one of the monkeys. Day 1 shows the effect of saline injection, with morphine self-administered at a low rate both before and after the injection. On Day 2, an injection of 0.1 mg/kg nalorphine produced no initial change in self-administration rate, but after 20 to 25 minutes a large increase in responding appeared which continued for 20 to 30 minutes. With repeated presentations of this dose of nalorphine, the appearance of increased self-administration responding occurred earlier. By Day 4, the increased rate of self-administration appeared within two minutes of the nalorphine injection. Similar results were seen with the other two monkeys. If it is assumed that the abstinence syndrome precipitated by nalorphine is aversive and that morphine decreases the aversiveness of the nalorphine-induced abstinence, then the decreased response latencies following nalorphine injections may reflect the development of conditioned escape responding.

After testing for the US properties of nalorphine, conditioning training was begun. A stimulus (flashing red light) was illuminated once a day for 10 minutes before and 30 minutes after an intravenous injection of saline. Following four light-saline injection pairings (Days 1 to 4), an intravenous injection of 0.1 mg/kg nalorphine was substituted for the saline (Days 5 to 14). After ten light-nalorphine injection pairing, followed by five days of test trials (Days 16 to 20), with light-saline injection pairings. Reconditioning training, with additional light-nalorphine injection pairings, was conducted on Days 21 to 30, followed by additional test trials on Days 32 to 35. The procedure is summarized in Table 1.

Table 1. *Procedure for conditioning changes in morphine self-administration behavior.*

DAY	1-4	5-14	15	16-20	21-30	31	32-35
LIGHT-INJECTION PAIRING	LIGHT + SALINE	LIGHT + NALORPHINE	NONE	LIGHT + SALINE	LIGHT + NALORPHINE	NONE	LIGHT + SALINE

Figure 2 shows the change in the frequency of morphine self-administration in the 30-minute period following injection of saline or nalorphine. No

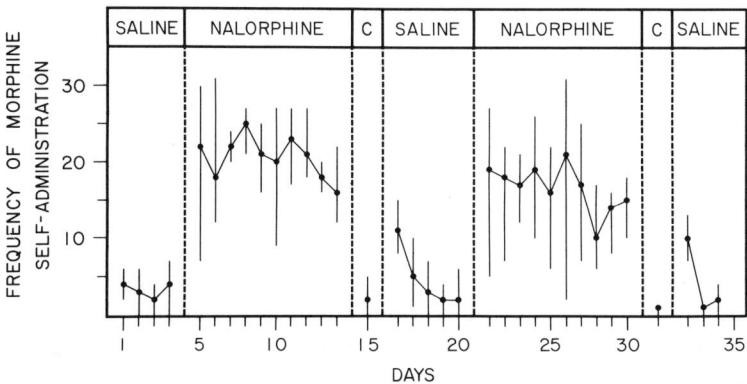

Fig. 2. Morphine self-administration during 30-min period after intravenous injection of saline or 0.1 mg/kg nalorphine. Each point represents the average frequency of self-administration for three morphine-dependent monkeys; vertical bars represent the range. No injection of saline or nalorphine was administered on the control day (c) following acquisition and reacquisition training. (From Goldberg, Woods, and Schuster, 1969. Science, 166:1306-1307. Copyright 1969 by the American Association for the Advancement of Science.)

change in the number of morphine self-administrations was produced by initial saline injection (Days 1 to 4). During conditioning trials (Days 5 to 14), intravenous injection of 0.1 mg/kg nalorphine produced large increases in the number of morphine self-administrations in the 30-minute period following the injection. After the tenth conditioning trial, a control day (Day 15) with no injection of saline or nalorphine yielded a self-administration rate similar to earlier light-saline injection levels (Days 1 to 4), indicating that the conditioning procedure had not interfered with baseline operant performance. The first test presentation of a red light-saline injection pairing (Day 16) resulted in large increases in the number of morphine self-administrations during the 30-minute period following the saline injection. The self-administration rate of the three monkeys was three to four times greater than that seen following the initial light-saline injection trials (Days 1 to 4). With repeated light-saline injection pairings (Days 16 to 20), this conditioned response rapidly disappeared. Reconditioning training produced results similar to those of the initial conditioning sessions. No change in self-administration responding was seen during the 10-minute interval between light onset and injections of saline or nalorphine.

Discussion. The finding that the rate of morphine responding increased to the saline-injection CS, though not the light CS, indicates that the interoceptive stimuli associated with the injection procedure had come to control, to some extent, the animal's behavior. This is consistent with similar observations by Goldberg, Woods, and Schuster (1968) indicating conditioned nalorphine-like responses to saline injections and with findings of Schuster and Brady (1964), that saline injections have discriminative stimulus properties. Recently, Schuster and Woods (1968) demonstrated that the intravenous injection procedure can also become part of a conditioned stimulus complex associated with intravenous morphine reinforcement in rhesus monkeys. During extinction of morphine self-administration responding, the response-contingent presentation of this stimulus complex produced large increases in response rate previously maintained by morphine reinforcement. Thus, stimuli associated with either the nalorphine-induced abstinence syndrome or with morphine reinforcement can become conditioned stimuli capable of influencing operant morphine self-administration behavior.

Wikler (1965) has suggested that relapse to drug-taking behavior is due to the failure of treatment programs to extinguish conditioned environmental stimuli associated with previous episodes of abstinence and their relief by opioid self-administration. When patients are allowed to return to their home environment after treatment, these conditioned stimuli may precipitate abstinence changes which have been relieved in the past by drug-taking behavior. If such behavior has not been extinguished during treatment, the patient responds to these abstinence changes as during dependence by self-administering the drug. This hypothesis is supported by the present finding that conditioned stimuli associated with the morphine-abstinence syndrome can produce large increases in drug-taking behavior.

CONDITIONED CHANGES IN FOOD-REINFORCED BEHAVIOR AND PHYSIOLOGIC RESPONSES

Method and Results. Five rhesus monkeys (*Macaca mulatta*), maintained by subcutaneous injections of 2 to 3 mg/kg morphine sulfate every six hours for at least two months, were surgically prepared with chronic jugular catheters (Schuster and Brady, 1964) and placed on a chain schedule of reinforcement involving a 30-minute fixed-interval component, producing a 60-minute fixed-ratio ten (FR-10) food-reinforcement component, followed by a 30-minute time-out component. For purposes of this chapter, however, only the FR 10 food component will be considered. The animals were run on this schedule for two hours each day, one to two hours after their last morphine injection.

After performance stabilized, drug conditioning training was begun. Five days of adaptation training were given (Days 1 to 5) in which an external conditioned stimulus (tone or red light) was aperiodically presented every third or fourth food-reinforcement session, approximately 10 minutes after the start of the FR 10 component, for 5 minutes before and after an intravenous injection of 1 ml saline. Ten days of acquisition training (Days 6 to 15) followed, in which the CS was presented as before but with intravenous injection of 0.2 mg/kg nalorphine (US) substituted for saline. Control sessions (no CS-injection pairing) were interspersed with days of adaptation and acquisition training. (For a more complete description of this see Goldberg and Schuster, 1967, 1970.)

An intravenous injection of 0.2 mg/kg nalorphine (US) produced immediate suppression of food-reinforced FR responding, as well as physiologic changes indicative of morphine abstinence syndrome in morphine-dependent monkeys. These unconditioned responses for all animals included a suppression of food responding, an increase in heart rate to 240-260 beats/min from an average during the food period of 185 beats/min, an increase in respiratory rate to 40-60 per minute, from an average during the food period of 20 per minute, an average decrease in respiration amplitude of 50 percent, a fall in body temperature of 1° to 2° C, vomiting and excessive salivation.

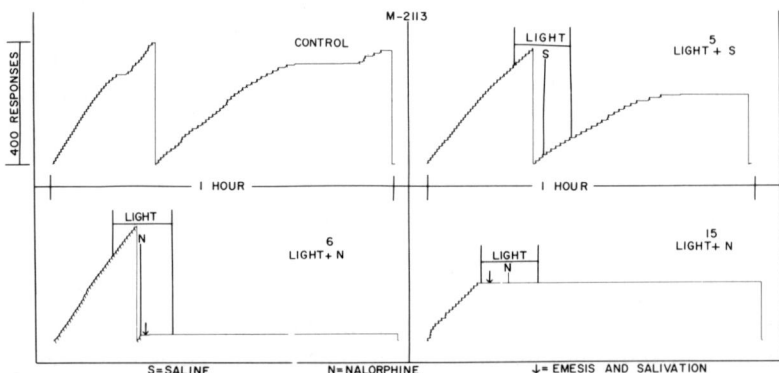

Fig. 3. The development of conditioned behavioral changes to nalorphine as indicated by cumulative response records of selected sessions for Monkey M2113. Each segment shows responding on a FR-10 schedule for food reinforcement. *Control:* Session before CS (light)-injection pairings. *5:* Initial absence of response to red light paired with saline injection. *6:* First acquisition session showing unconditioned effects of nalorphine on food responding. *15:* Tenth acquisition session showing conditioned response to CS (light). Arrows indicate emesis and excessive salivation. (Modified from Goldberg and Schuster, 1970.)

Figure 3 shows cumulative response records of selected sessions during adaptation and acquisition for one monkey. In control sessions prior to conditioning training, more prolonged pausing after reinforcement was found than is usually seen on this type of schedule, but performance over sessions was stable. Session 5 was the final adaptation session. The onset of the red light and saline injection caused no disruption in food-reinforced responding. Session 6 was the first acquisition session with light-nalorphine injection (CS-US) pairing. The monkey responded normally during the CS period before the nalorphine injection. Responding was completely suppressed after the nalorphine injection and continued suppressed for the remainder of the session. Vomiting and excessive salivation, indicated by arrows in Figure 3, were also seen after the nalorphine injection. Session 15, the tenth acquisition session with CS-US pairing, illustrates conditioned suppression of food responding. Prior to the CS onset, the monkey's food response rate was comparable to control days. With the onset of the CS, however, food responding was almost completely suppressed and continued so for the remainder of the session. In Session 15, conditioned vomiting and salivation were also observed during the 5-minute CS period prior to nalorphine injection.

Figure 4 shows the average percent change in food response rate from the 5-minute period preceding the CS onset to the 5-minute period during

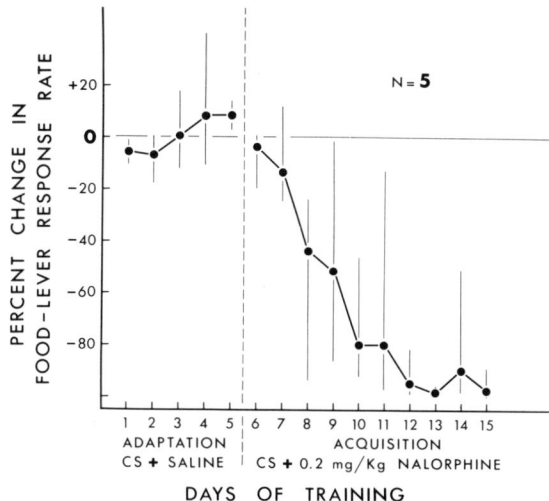

Fig. 4. Percent change in food response rate from the 5-min period preceding onset of CS (tone or red light) to the 5-min period during CS presentation and before injection of saline, or 0.2 mg/kg nalorphine (CS-US interval). Points represent average percent change in response rate of five monkeys; vertical bars represent the range. Each acquisition session was followed by 2 to 3 control sessions not indicated on the graph. (Based on combined data from Goldberg and Schuster, 1967, 1970.)

the CS and before the injection of nalorphine or saline (CS-US interval). Figure 5 shows the average percent change in heart rate during the same periods. During adaptation (Days 1 to 5), no change was seen in either food-reinforced responding or heart rate during the 5-minute CS-US interval. After the second acquisition trial (Day 7), response rate during the CS-US interval decreased, and was almost completely suppressed after the fourth acquisition trial (Day 9). After the third acquisition trial (Day 8), heart rate during the 5-minute CS-US interval decreased, and a maximal decrease in heart rate was reached following the fourth acquisition session. All five monkeys showed the conditioned suppression of food responding, but two of the five monkeys showed no change in heart rate at any time during acquisition, except after nalorphine injections. Two monkeys showed vomiting and excessive salivation during the CS-US interval on acquisition trials 7 to 10 (Days 12 to 15). No change in respiratory rate, respiration amplitude, or temperature was seen in any of the monkeys during acquisition, except after injections of nalorphine.

Discussion. The decrease in food-reinforced behavior produced by nalorphine in morphine-dependent monkeys agrees with observations by Thompson and Schuster (1964) that abstinence induced by morphine depri-

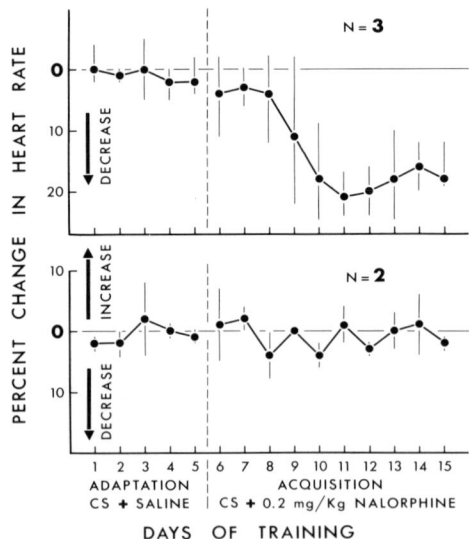

Fig. 5. Percent change in heart rate from the 5-min period preceding the onset of the CS (tone or red light) to the 5-min period during CS presentation and before injection of saline, or 0.2 mg/kg nalorphine (CS-US interval). The upper graph shows adaptation (1 to 5) and acquisition (6 to 15) sessions for three of five monkeys with conditioned heart-rate changes. The lower graph shows adaptation (1 to 5) and acquisition (6 to 15) sessions for two monkeys that failed to demonstrate conditioned heart-rate changes. Points represent the average percent change in heart rate; vertical bars represent the range. Each acquisition session was followed by 2 to 3 control sessions not indicated on the graph. (Based on combined data from Goldberg and Schuster, 1967, 1970).

vation results in a similar decrease. Suppression of food-reinforced behavior conditioned more rapidly than changes in heart rate. Similar results have been found with rats (de Toledo and Black, 1966; Parrish, 1967) using the CER paradigm with electric shock. Conditioning of vomiting and salivation developed more slowly than either food-response suppression or heart rate changes.

While the heart-rate response to nalorphine was always an increase, the response to the CS was usually a decrease. These findings are consistent with those of de Toledo and Black (1966), Parrish (1967), and Brady (1967), using the CER paradigm with electric shock, and with numerous classical discrimination conditioning studies (Schneiderman, Smith, Smith, and Gormezano, 1966; Schneiderman, Vandercar, Yehle, Manning, and Schneiderman, 1969; Yehle, Dauth, and Schneiderman, 1967). The findings do not agree with those of Stebbins and Smith (1964) or Nathan and Smith (1968). These latter authors found the response to the CS to be an increase in heart rate, rather than the decrease found in the present experiments. It is possible that, in the present experiment, a five-minute average of heart rate would obscure any increases that may have been of short duration. This possibility can be excluded since the simultaneous measurement of beat-to-beat heart rate obtained from tachograph recordings showed no rate increase. The decrease in heart rate was slow in onset, the predominant decrease occurring in the last two to three minutes of the CS-US interval. At the present time, there is not sufficient information available to account for the recorded differences in direction during heart rate conditioning.

A possible explanation for the decrease in heart rate is that it is an indirect result of the suppression in food responding. Before trial sessions with saline or nalorphine administration, however, monkeys occasionally ceased responding for food on the FR 10 schedule but heart rate remained at a level of 170 to 190 beats/min. The failure to see conditioned heart-rate changes in two of the monkeys and the difference in speed of acquisition of conditioned changes in food responding and heart rate further argues against such an explanation. Using a similar paradigm with rats and electric shock, de Toledo and Black (1966) found conditioning of food-response suppression and heart-rate decreases to proceed relatively independently. Goldberg and Schuster (1967) suggested that the conditioned physiologic changes (emesis, salivation, and heart rate decrease) could be responsible for disrupting the monkeys' food-reinforced behavior. This explanation was no longer tenable, however, after experiments with additional monkeys were conducted (Goldberg and Schuster, 1970). Two of five monkeys studied showed no conditioned physiologic changes, and conditioned emesis and salivation were observed with only two of the five monkeys, additional evidence that conditioning of the different responses proceeds relatively independently.

SITUATIONAL CONDITIONING

In the preceding experiments (Goldberg and Schuster, 1967, 1969), three monkeys exhibited what appeared to be conditioned nalorphine responses to the experimental situation during control sessions following the fifth, sixth, eighth, and ninth acquisition sessions. Although neither the light or tone CS nor injection was presented to these monkeys, response rate suppression, heart rate decreases, vomiting, and salivation were observed at approximately the same time that the CS and US would ordinarily have been presented. Such findings are consistent with early findings of Pavlov (1927) and with Estes' (1959) suggestion that animals become conditioned to the total stimulus complex. Figure 6 presents selected cumulative response records for two of the monkeys showing this response. Session 1, a control session prior to the sixth acquisition trial, shows no disruption of food-reinforced responding. Session 2, the first control session following the sixth acquisition trial, shows suppression of responding, vomiting, and salivation. By the control session on the following day (Session 3), however, these responses had disappeared.

The role of generalization in abstinence-associated conditioning has not been investigated. However, the appearance of conditioned responses to the experimental situation, in the absence of the specific stimuli utilized for acquisition training, suggests that such conditioning could exist in the less rigidly controlled environment of the human narcotic user.

EXTINCTION OF CONDITIONING IN MORPHINE-DEPENDENT MONKEYS

The conditioned nalorphine response of two monkeys (M474 and M574) was extinguished with daily pairings of the CS and saline injection, during which time the animals were maintained on chronic morphine treatment (Goldberg and Schuster, 1967). Both animals previously showed conditioned suppression of food responding, and one of these animals (M574) showed conditioned heart rate decrease, vomiting, and excessive salivation, as well.

For M574, the conditioned vomiting and salivation were extinguished after ten extinction sessions, whereas the heart rate response was only partially extinguished after 15 sessions and food responding remained completely suppressed. Food responding continued to be suppressed for another 13 sessions.

For M474, after 10 extinction sessions, food response rate approached normal baseline levels during CS, but occasionally suppression occurred. To hasten complete extinction, the FR requirement was reduced during the CS period and then gradually returned to FR 10 over the next eight to nine sessions. Response rates during the CS increased over these sessions to a value approximating that of the initial adaptation sessions. Reacquisition sessions pairing CS and 0.2 mg/kg nalorphine injection were then conducted, with results closely paralleling those of the initial conditioning sessions. For a more detailed presentation of these results, see Goldberg and Schuster (1967).

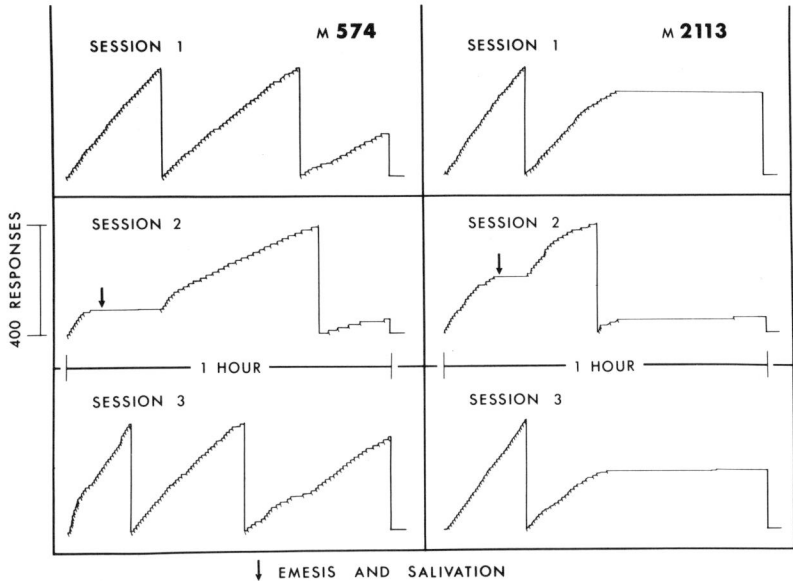

Fig. 6. Conditioned nalorphine response to the situational complex. Cumulative response records for Monkeys M574 and M2113. *Session 1:* Control session prior to the sixth acquisition trial. *Session 2:* First control session following the sixth acquisition trial. *Session 3:* Second control session after the sixth acquisition trial. Arrows indicate emesis and excessive salivation. (Based on combined data from Goldberg and Schuster, 1967, 1970.)

EXTINCTION OF CONDITIONING IN POST-DEPENDENT MONKEYS

Method and Results. For two monkeys showing a conditioned nalorphine response, the chronic morphine treatment was abruptly discontinued (Goldberg and Schuster, 1970). To determine the persistency of the conditioned food-response suppression and change in heart rate, following long periods of morphine deprivation, the monkeys were tested at monthly intervals for one to four months with CS (red light)-saline injection pairings.

Figures 7 and 8 show cumulative response records of the two monkeys (M2115 and M2116) extinguished in this manner. Control, adaptation (Session 5), and acquisition (Sessions 6 and 15) training effects were similar to those described earlier. The chronic morphine treatment of both monkeys

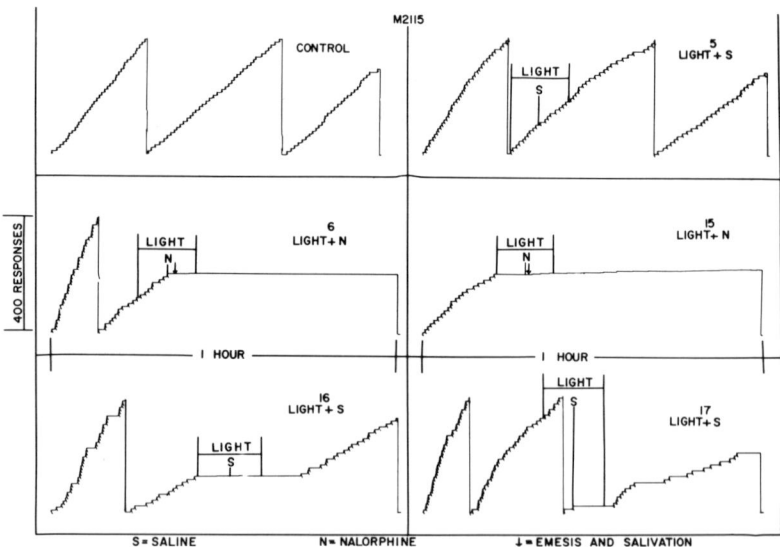

Fig. 7. Cumulative response records of selected sessions for Monkey M2115, showing development and persistence of conditioned behavioral changes. *Control:* Session before CS (red light)-injection pairings. *5:* Last adaptation session. *6:* First acquisition session. *15:* Tenth acquisition session. *16 and 17:* Monthly test sessions for the persistence of the light and saline injection as conditioned stimuli following cessation of chronic morphine treatment. Arrows indicate emesis and excessive salivation. (Modified from Goldberg and Schuster, 1970.)

was discontinued following Session 15. Session 16 was the first session with CS-saline injection presentation 30 days after morphine deprivation. As can be seen, the food responding of both monkeys was almost completely suppressed throughout the entire CS period. Session 17 was the second session with CS-saline presentation, conducted 60 days after the termination of chronic morphine treatment. The food responding of M2116 was completely suppressed throughout the CS period, while that of M2115 failed to be suppressed with onset of the CS. Following the saline injection, however, responding of M2115 was suppressed for the remaining five minutes of the CS period. Monkey M2116 continued to show complete suppression of food responding on the 90th and 120th day after termination of chronic morphine treatment.

In Acquisition Sessions 11 to 15, for M2115, heart rate declined during the five-minute CS-US interval. No heart changes were observed in M2116 during the CS-US interval. After injection of nalorphine, heart rate of both monkeys increased from a normal FR 10 food period level of 180-210 beats/min to 240-260 beats/min. In Sessions 16 and 17, after 30 and 60 days

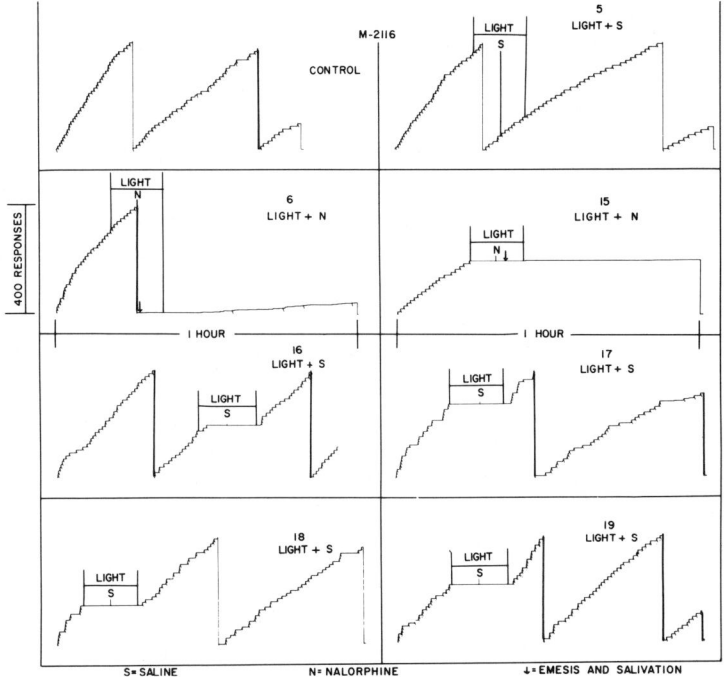

Fig. 8. Cumulative response records of selected sessions for Monkey M2116, showing development and persistence of conditioned behavioral changes. *Control:* Session before CS (red light)-injection pairings. *5:* Last adaptation session. *6:* First acquisition session. *15:* Tenth acquisition session. *16 to 19:* Monthly test sessions for persistence of the light and saline injection as conditioned stimuli following cessation of chronic morphine treatment. Arrows indicate emesis and excessive salivation. (Modified from Goldberg and Schuster, 1970.)

of morphine deprivation, the heart rate of M2115 again decreased during the CS period.

No vomiting, excessive salivation, nor changes in respiration or temperature were observed in M2115 or M2116 during the CS periods preceding any of the injections. In the five-minute period following the injection of nalorphine, both monkeys showed emesis, excessive salivation, an increase in respiratory rate from 15 to 25 per minute to 40 to 60, a decrease in respiratory amplitude of approximately 50 percent, and an average fall in temperature of 1°C from a normal FR 10 food period level of 38° to 39°C. At no time in the experiment was any change seen in the form of the EKG.

Following Session 17 for M2115 and Session 19 for M2116, repeated presentations of the CS-saline injection complex led to the extinction of the conditioned suppression of food responding and conditioned heart rate changes. Nevertheless, conditioned suppression could be rapidly reinstated by additional nalorphine injections.

Discussion. The hypothesis that conditioning factors are important motivating factors in the relapse of post-dependent subjects to drug-taking behavior is supported by the finding of Goldberg, Woods, and Schuster (1969), that CS associated with the nalorphine-induced abstinence syndrome are capable of producing large increases in drug-taking behavior. The hypothesis is further supported by the finding of Goldberg and Schuster (1970), that the CS developed by association with the nalorphine-induced abstinence syndrome retain their ability to elicit conditioned behavioral and physiologic changes after two to four months of morphine deprivation, when animals are no longer physically dependent on morphine. The persistence of conditioned changes, similar to those described in these studies, could be a major motivating factor in the relapse of patients to drug use after treatment. For a more extensive review of the literature concerning the relationship of conditioning to relapse, and a detailed discussion of the implications for treatment programs, see Goldberg (1970).

The long-lasting persistence of conditioned changes associated with the morphine-abstinence syndrome, after prolonged periods of morphine deprivation, agrees with the results obtained by Wikler and Pescor (1967) with rats and demonstrates that the persistence of the behavioral and physiologic changes conditioned in the preceding experiments is not entirely dependent on the drug state of the animals.

RECONDITIONING NALORPHINE EFFECTS IN POST-DEPENDENT MONKEYS

When conditioned nalorphine changes are completely extinguished, after two to four months deprivation, conditioning can be rapidly reinstated by additional nalorphine injections (Goldberg and Schuster, 1970). These results are shown in selected cumulative response records for M2115 (Figure 9) and for M2116 (Figure 10). A control session, which followed the final extinction session with a light-saline injection pairing, is shown for each monkey. As can be seen, food responding was stable and at normal rates, indicating the conditioning and extinction procedures had not interfered with the baseline FR performance. In the final extinction session (Session 28 for M2115, Session 25 for M2116) light-saline injection presentation failed to disrupt food responding. The intravenous administration of 0.2 mg/kg of nalorphine in the first reacquisition session (Session 29 for M2115, Session 26 for M2116) immediately suppressed food-reinforced FR behavior

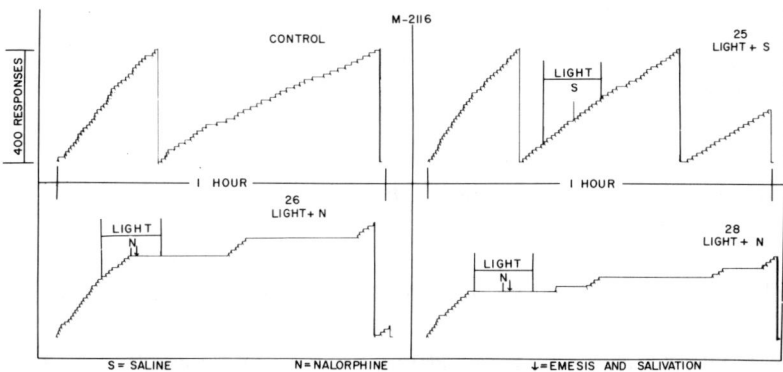

Fig. 9. Cumulative response records of selected sessions for Monkey M2115, showing the extinction and reacquisition of conditioned behavioral changes after 60 days of morphine abstinence. *Control:* Session before reacquisition sessions with CS (red light)-nalorphine pairings. *28:* Last extinction session prior to reacquisition. *29:* First reacquisition session. *31:* Third reacquisition session. Arrows indicate emesis and excessive salivation. (Modified from Goldberg and Schuster 1970.)

and produced vomiting and excessive salivation (indicated by arrows in Figures 9 and 10). Food responding of both monkeys remained suppressed for the remainder of the session.

After two pairings of CS and nalorphine injection (Session 31 for M2115, Session 28 for M2116), the onset of CS again produced complete

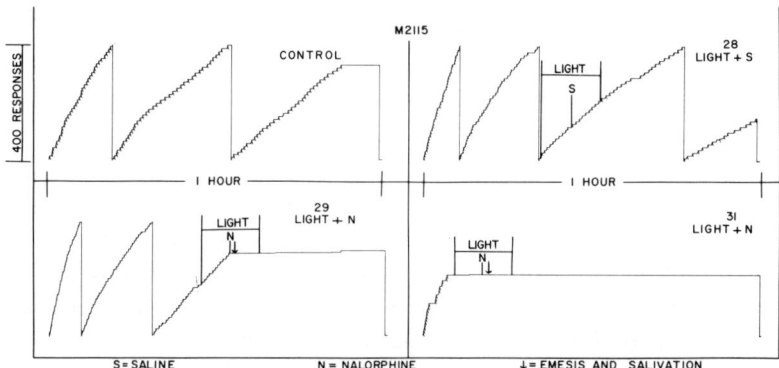

Fig. 10. Cumulative response records of selected sessions for Monkey M2116, showing the extinction and reacquisition of conditioned behavioral changes after 120 days of morphine abstinence. *Control:* Session before reacquisition sessions with CS (red light)-nalorphine pairings. *25:* Last extinction session prior to reacquisition. *26:* First reacquisition session. *28:* Third reacquisition session. Arrows indicate emesis and excessive salivation. (Modified from Goldberg and Schuster, 1970.)

suppression of food responding in both monkeys, and a decrease in heart rate of M2115 (not shown in these figures). Similar results with nalorphine in post-dependent monkeys, described earlier, were found by Irwin and Seevers (1956). It is not clear whether the altered response to nalorphine in the post-dependent monkey is a conditioned response resulting from prior experience with nalorphine-induced abstinence, or an unconditioned response resulting from a persistent, residual, physiologic change in the monkey following a period of chronic morphine treatment.

SENSITIVITY OF POST-DEPENDENT MONKEYS TO NALORPHINE

Method and Results. In an attempt to determine whether post-dependent monkeys, with no previous history of nalorphine-induced abstinence, have an altered sensitivity to nalorphine, three monkeys, previously maintained for two months on 12 mg/kg/day morphine sulfate, were completely deprived of morphine for three months and trained on an FR 10 food reinforcement schedule (Goldberg and Schuster, 1969). The schedule was identical to that described earlier. These monkeys had never experienced nalorphine-induced abstinence while dependent on morphine, nor received nalorphine prior to this study. After four saline control sessions, a range of nalorphine doses was administed in ascending order over successive days during the FR 10 food reinforcement period. Two monkeys never exposed to morphine were tested for their sensitivity to nalorphine in the same way. All injections were intravenous through a chronically implanted catheter.

The percent change in food response rate, from the five-minute period preceding injection of saline or different doses of nalorphine, to the five-minute period following the injection of saline or nalorphine, is shown for the five monkeys in Figure 11. Doses of nalorphine, from 0.2 mg/kg to 1.6 mg/kg, produced no change in food responding for the two normal monkeys as compared to saline control levels. Not until a dose of 3.2 mg/kg of nalorphine was reached was suppression of their food responding observed. The three post-dependent monkeys showed no change in their response rate after doses of nalorphine from 0.1 to 0.4 mg/kg. Unlike the normal monkeys, however, the 0.8 and 1.6 mg/kg doses of nalorphine suppressed food responding. A dose of 3.2 mg/kg of nalorphine, which only partially suppressed the food response rate of normal monkeys, almost completely suppressed responding of the three post-dependent monkeys. In addition, vomiting, excessive salivation, and hyperirritability were observed in the three post-dependent monkeys after the 3.2 and 6.4 mg/kg injections of nalorphine. This was not seen with the normal monkeys.

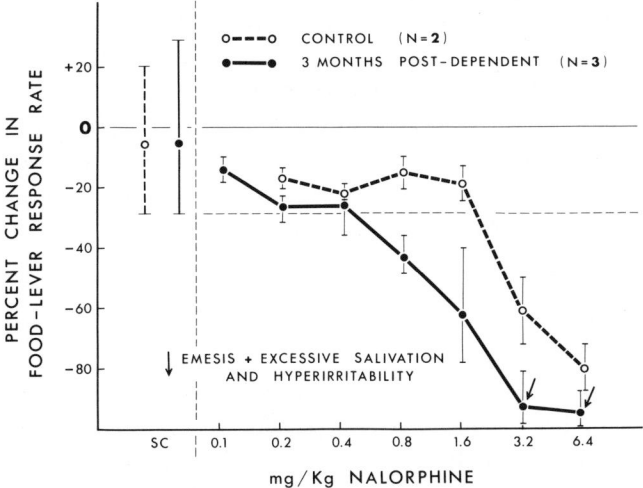

Fig. 11. Average percent change in food-lever response rate from the 5-min period preceding intravenous injection of saline or nalorphine to the 5-min period following injection of saline or nalorphine. The two far left points represent the average, and the brackets the range, of four saline control (SC) sessions. The horizontal dotted line indicates the lower limit of the range on saline control sessions. At each of the doses of nalorphine the points represent the average percent change in food-lever response rate and the brackets represent the range. Arrows indicate emesis, excessive salivation, and hyperirritability. (From Goldberg and Schuster, 1969. Science, 166:1548-1549. Copyright 1969 by the American Association for the Advancement of Science.)

Discussion. These findings indicate that post-dependent (morphine) rhesus monkeys have an increased sensitivity to nalorphine that appears to be the result of long-lasting physiologic changes and not the result of previous conditioning. Other investigators have demonstrated that a period of chronic exposure to morphine in man, or exposure to a single dose of morphine in rats, results in a significant degree of tolerance (decreased sensitivity) to morphine several months later (Cochin and Kornetsky, 1964; Fraser and Isbell, 1952; Kornetsky and Bain, 1968). In studies of physical dependence produced by a number of drugs in both animals and man (Himmelsbach, 1942; Martin, 1967; Martin, Wikler, Eades, and Pescor, 1963), certain signs of the abstinence syndrome have been shown to persist for many months and have been called a secondary abstinence syndrome (Martin et al., 1963). Altered sensitivity to nalorphine, morphine, and perhaps other drugs may be an important aspect of this secondary abstinence syndrome.

It should be noted that nalorphine failed to produce any changes in food-lever responding at the dose level used for the present conditioning studies (0.2 mg/kg). This would indicate that the sensitivity of Monkeys M2115 and M2116 to nalorphine, after two to four months of morphine deprivation, is primarily a conditioned effect related to the previous conditioning history of the animals, which included repeated experience with the nalorphine-induced abstinence syndrome. The persistence of physiologic changes, resulting in increased sensitivity to nalorphine's effects, may have facilitated this conditioning by making the animals more sensitive to the stimulus properties of nalorphine.

SUMMARY

This chapter describes a procedure developed to study the classical conditioning of both behavioral and physiologic aspects of the morphine-abstinence syndrome in the physically dependent rhesus monkey. The experiments reviewed demonstrate the usefulness of the procedure in a critical analysis of the conditioned components of narcotic dependence. The similarity between the results obtained using nalorphine as the US and other studies using similar paradigms with electric shock illustrates the application of the techniques of classical conditioning to the study of drugs.

REFERENCES

Brady, J.V. Emotion and the sensitivity of psychoendocrine systems. In D.C. Glass, ed., *Neurophysiology and Emotion.* New York, The Rockefeller University Press, 1967, 70.

Cochin, J., and Kornetsky, C. Development and loss of tolerance to morphine in the rat after single and multiple injections. *J. Pharmacol. Exp. Ther.*, 1964, *145*, 1.

Deneau, G.A., and Seevers, M.H. Pharmacological aspects of drug dependence. *Advances Pharmacol.*, 1964, *3*, 267.

────── Yanagita, T., and Seevers, M.H. Intravenous narcotic self-administration procedures in primates. *Psychopharmacologia*, 1969, *11*.

de Toledo, L., and Black, A.H. Heart Rate: Changes during conditioned suppression in rats. *Science*, 1966, *152*, 1404.

Eddy, N.B., Halbach, H., Isbell, H., and Seevers, M.H. Drug Dependence: Its significance and characteristics. *Bull. WHO*, 1965, *32*, 721.

Estes, W.K. The statistical approach to learning theory. In S. Koch, ed., *Psychology: A Study of a Science.* New York, McGraw-Hill Book Company, 1959, *2*, 380.

────── and Skinner, B.F. Some quantitative properties of anxiety. *J. Exp. Psychol.*, 1941, *29*, 390.

Fraser, H.F., and Isbell, H. Comparative effects of 20 mg of morphine sulfate on non-adicts and former morphine addicts. *J. Pharmacol. Exp. Ther.*, 1952, *105*, 498.

Goldberg, S.R. Relapse to opioid dependence: The role of conditioning. *Advances in Mental Science*, 1970, *2*.

────── and Schuster, C.R. Classical conditioning of the morphine-withdrawal syndrome. *Fed. Proc.*, 1966, *25*, 261. (Abstract)

—— and Schuster, C.R. Conditioned suppression by a stimulus associated with nalorphine in morphine-dependent monkeys. *J. Exp. Anal. Behav.*, 1967, *10*, 235.
—— and Schuster, C.R. Nalorphine: Increased sensitivity of monkeys formerly dependent on morphine. *Science*, 1969, *166*, 1548.
—— and Schuster, C.R. Conditioned nalorphine-induced abstinence changes: Persistence in post morphine-dependent monkeys. *J. Exp. Anal. Behav.*, 1970, *14*, 33.
—— Woods, J.H., and Schuster, C.R. Morphine: Conditioned increases in self-administration in rhesus monkeys. *Science*, 1969, *166*, 1306.
—— Woods, J.H., and Schuster, C.R. Nalorphine-induced changes in morphine self-administration in rhesus monkeys. *Fed. Proc.*, 1968, *27*, 754. (Abstract)
Himmselsbach, C.K. Clinical studies of drug addiction. Physical dependence, withdrawal and recovery. *Arch. Intern. Med.*, 1942, *69*, 766.
Irwin, S., and Seevers, M.H. Comparative study of regular and N-allylnormorphine induced withdrawal in monkeys addicted to morphine, 6-methyldihydromorphine, Dromoran, methadone and ketobemidone. *J. Pharmacol. Exp. Ther.*, 1952, *106*, 397. (Abstract)
—— and Seevers, M.H. Altered response to drugs in the post addict (Macaca mulatta). *J. Pharmacol. Exp. Ther.*, 1956, *116*, 31. (Abstract)
Jaffe, J. Narcotic Analgesics. In L.S. Goodman and A. Gilman, eds., *The Pharmacological Basis of Therapeutics*, 3rd ed. New York, The Macmillan Company, 1965, 247.
Kornetsky, C., and Bain, G. Morphine: Single-dose tolerance. *Science*, 1968, *162*, 1011.
Martin, W.R. Opioid antagonists. *Pharmacol. Rev.*, 1967, *19*, 463.
—— Wikler, A., Eades, C.G., and Pescor, F.T. Tolerance to and physical dependence on morphine in rats. *Psychopharmacologia*, 1963, *4*, 247.
Nathan, M.A., and Smith, O.A., Jr. Differential conditional emotional and cardiovascular responses—a training technique for monkeys. *J. Exp. Anal. Behav.*, 1968, *11*, 77.
Parrish, J. Classical discrimination conditioning of heart rate and bar-press suppression in the rat. *Psychonomic Science*, 1967, *9*, 267.
Pavlov, I.P. *Conditional Reflex*. Trans. and ed. by G.V. Anrep. London, Oxford University Press, 1927.
Razran, G. Avoidant vs unavoidant conditioning and partial reinforcement in Russian laboratories. *Amer. J. Psychol.*, 1956, *69*, 127.
Reynolds, W.F. Acquisition and extinction of the conditioned eyelid response following partial and continuous reinforcement. *J. Exp. Psychol.*, 1958, *55*, 335.
Schneiderman, N., Smith, M.C., Smith, A.C., and Gormezano, I. Heart rate classical conditioning in rabbits. *Psychonomic Science*, 1966, *6*, 241.
—— Vandercar, D.H., Yehle, A.L., Manning, A.A., Golden, T., and Schneiderman, E. Vagal compensatory adjustment: Relationship to heart rate classical conditioning in rabbits. *J. Comp. Physiol. Psychol.*, 1969, *68*, 175.
Schuster, C.R., and Brady, J.V. The discriminative control of a food-reinforced operant by interoceptive stimulation. *Pavlov Journal of Higher Nervous Activity*, 1964, *14*, 448.
—— and Thompson, T. Self-administration of drugs. *Ann. Rev. Pharmacol.*, 1969, *9*, 483.
—— and Woods, J.H. The conditioned reinforcing effects of stimuli associated with morphine reinforcement. *International Journal of the Addictions*, 1968, *3*, 223.
Stebbins, W.C., and Smith, O.A., Jr. Cardiovascular concomitants of the conditioned emotional response in the monkey. *Science*, 1964, *144*, 881.
Thompson, T., and Schuster, C.R. Morphine self-administration, food-reinforced, and avoidance behaviors in rhesus monkeys. *Psychopharmacology*, 1964, *5*, 87.
Weeks, J.R., and Collins, R.J. Patterns of intravenous self-injection by morphine-addicted rats. *Res. Publ. Ass. Res. Nerv. Ment. Dis.*, 1968, *46*, 288.
Wikler, A. Conditioning factors in opiate addiction and relapse. In D.M. Wilner and G.G. Kassebaum, eds., *Narcotics*. New York, McGraw-Hill Book Company, 1965, 85.

—— and Pescor, F.T. Classical conditioning of a morphine abstinence phenomenon, reinforcement of opioid-drinking behavior and "relapse" in morphine-addicted rats. *Psychopharmacologia*, 1967, *10*, 255.

Woods, L.A. The pharmacology of nalorphine (N-allylnormorphine). *Pharmacol. Rev.*, 1956, *8*, 175.

Yanagita, T., Deneau, G.A., and Seevers, M.H. Evaluation of pharmacologic agents in the monkey by long-term intravenous self or programmed administration. *Excerpta Medica International Congress Series*, 1965, *87*, 453.

Yehle, A., Dauth, G., and Schneiderman, N. Correlates of heart-rate classical conditioning in curarized rabbits. *J. Comp. Physiol. Psychol.*, 1967, *64*, 98.

Unconditioned Stimulus Functions of Drugs: Interpretations. I

Howard F. Hunt

Department of Psychiatry
Columbia University
New York, New York

This volume as a whole emphasizes that drugs and their effects can be conceptualized analytically as "stimuli," having three important stimulus functions—eliciting, reinforcing, and discriminative functions. In their eliciting function, drugs can act as unconditioned stimuli in a Pavlovian or Type-S conditioning paradigm; that is, drug effects, paired with other stimuli in the Pavlovian mode, can endow those stimuli with new behavior-eliciting powers. This is not quite the same as saying, however, that only the responses elicited by the drug have been conditioned to the new stimulus, as Pavlovian conditioned responses, or that the conditioned changes that have taken place must be interpreted as exclusively Pavlovian.

Dr. Perez-Cruet (Chapter 2) reported on an intriguing series of experiments in which bulbocapnine injections during presentation of an auditory stimulus endowed it with the power to evoke changes in EKG form, heart rate, respiration, and (in two dogs) changes in motor activity similar to those produced by bulbocapnine. He pointed out that such conditioning could not be produced when the "unconditioned stimulus" was injection of a drug that evoked its responses through peripheral mechanisms (e.g., atropine in production of tachycardia); it required the involvement of the central nervous system in the sequence. (Here, though the data showed that central nervous system involvement was necessary to produce these conditioning effects, this should not be taken to prove that such involvement is sufficient. Differentia-

---

[1] Some of the suggestions as to mechanisms involved in conditioning of drug effects and dependency developed out of research conducted under USPHS Grant No. MH-07279.

tion between necessary and sufficient conditions is both important and difficult in this area, as in others.)

Then he went on to show how such Type-S conditioning techniques, with faradic shock as the unconditioned stimulus and using a refined beat-by-beat averaging of heart rate, could help clarify new details about the mechanisms of cardiac control and conditioning. He also combined the procedures with the administration of blocking agents such as propranolol to vagotomized and atropinized dogs to make a beginning on the functional dissection of these mechanisms.

The major interpretations in this paper appear to view the conditioning in the bulbocapnine and faradic-shock experiments only from the Pavlovian perspective, even though Dr. Perez-Cruet cautions that the conventional distinction between Pavlovian and instrumental conditioning may be too hard and fast and simplistic. If these two supposedly distinct kinds of behavioral processes cannot be considered as independent and separate as many textbook discussions imply, the design and interpretation of the Pavlovian experiments here might well have included more explicit concern with determining what response classes were, in fact, being conditioned.

This comment is intended not to explain away or detract from the author's data and suggestions, but rather to call attention to the fact that Type-S (Pavlovian) and Type-R (operant or instrumental) conditioning refer to two different procedures rather than to two kinds of behavior or processes. In operant conditioning, stimuli associated with reward or punishment acquire conditioned reinforcing powers through Pavlovian pairings embedded in the procedure, to play a major role in facilitating the acquisition of the behavior and sustaining it. Similarly, the influence of reward and punishment intrudes, on occasion, into some Pavlovian experimental arrangements. The situation is not entirely clear even in the exciting recent work demonstrating that visceral responses (e.g., heart rate) usually under Type-S control can be placed under Type-R control even though the responses ordinarily are not thought to be manipulable by reward and punishment. In many of these experiments, one wonders just what response(s) is (are) being conditioned—the heart rate by itself, or some more extensive and complex response pattern of which the visceral response is but one component.

The studies of operant control of visceral responses customarily use peripherally acting motor blocking agents such as curare or succinylcholine to insure that the visceral responses are not produced as *consequences* of skeletal muscle activity. This procedure does not rule out, however, the possibility that the visceral responses being studied are part of a total efferent response pattern, which normally includes integrated visceral *and* skeletal muscle components, that normally *is* under operant control. Here the curare simply could be blocking the expression of the skeletal muscle component of the pattern, leaving the visceral component for the experimenter to see and measure.

It seems reasonable to expect that stimuli of sufficient biologic importance to the subject to serve as reinforcers will generally evoke complex patterns of response. As unconditioned stimuli in a Pavlovian experiment, they probably evoke many reflexes; simultaneously, they should have rewarding or punishing functions (operant reinforcement) with respect to a broad range of adaptive, integrated reaction patterns that involve not only skeletal muscle but visceral responses as well. In the Perez-Cruet experiments, it is not entirely clear that we are dealing only with the Pavlovian conditioning of selected cardiac reflexes evoked directly by the unconditioned stimuli, or that the data should be viewed just on that basis.

The vagotomized, atropinized dog being conditioned to Pavlovian foot withdrawal with faradic shock is a preparation having many behavioral and physiologic facets not considered closely in the analysis. Similarly, the bulbocapnine injections may have operated as aversive (unpleasant) stimuli. The effects of injections on cardiac function were brief (usually less than fifteen minutes in duration) while the catalepsy lasted for several hours. Perhaps the induction of catalepsy was very frightening when combined with isolation and the restrictions on escape imposed by the apparatus leads. We get so little description of overt behavior and so little by way of control observations that we cannot tell for sure whether the cardiac conditioning was direct, or implicated in a more general aversively conditioned response pattern. The consequences of such alternative possibilities were not considered in the interpretation, yet they could have important implications for the ultimate meaning of this work.

We are indebted to Pickens and Dougherty (Chapter 3) for their clear demonstration that activity changes following drug injections can come under the control of previously neutral stimuli as a result of pairing the two in a Pavlovian fashion. This clarity is a welcome improvement on the earlier work in this area, and shows the benefits to be reaped from taking the extra trouble to develop good procedures and designs.

I share their doubts about explanations of the effect based on habituation. The explanations are inherently ambiguous unless what is being habituated to what, and the effects such habituation produces on behavior, are clearly specified. Usually they are not; often they cannot be. We need to know whether habituation (inferred from exposure of the animal to the apparatus without reinforcement or new stimulation) has the same effect on behavior in the Y-maze, running wheel, and activity cage, and whether different drugs have differential effects on the process in each. In addition, the relationship between activity and habituation or novelty is probably an inverted U-shaped curve. Too much novelty immobilizes the rat with fear, while too little (as in habituation) results in very low levels of exploration and an inactive animal. Happily, just the right amount produces an active, exploring rat. The problem is to determine where the rat starts on this curve, and which way habituation under the drug or habituation under saline or direct drug effects move it. As these are among the facts we may be trying to discover with the experiment, the approach obviously leaves much to be desired.

We also share concerns about whether the control over activity established by the Pickens and Dougherty procedure is of the Type-S or Type-R variety. The procedure was Type-S, but this did not rule out possibilities of some sort of operant reinforcement for activity. They did not spell out these possibilities in any detail, but only suggested that the conditioned drug effect could represent nothing more than increased activity such as commonly appears upon presentation of a stimulus that signals the presentation of positive reinforcers (a property possessed by all the drugs that have been used to condition activity). Actually, a repetition of their injection experiments, but with an activity-reducing rather than a stimulating drug, might clarify this situation materially.

As a speculative alternative, it may be that the stimulus control here is discriminative rather than classically Pavlovian, and that the stimuli paired with receiving the drug, or arising from the direct actions of the drug, become discriminative stimuli for increased activity. The increased overall activity produced directly by the drug also increases the density (frequency) of those reinforcements (which are independent of the drug) that ordinarily maintain and support whatever behavior the animals emit in the activity cage. Behavior such as exploring, scratching, sniffing, rearing up, and the like probably are under at least partial control by Type-R reinforcement, even though the reinforcers cannot be identified very precisely at present. Thus, drug-produced stimuli, and stimuli paired with them, would be the occasions for increases in the reinforced occurrence of activity. To the extent that all this is so, behaviorally active drugs could acquire discriminative powers, however fortuitously or adventitiously. Such adventitious discriminative effects could represent one of the most durable conditioned consequences of drug administration, durable because the differential reinforcement of the discrimination depends only upon the continuation of reinforcement contingencies that are incorporated into the animal's ordinary living arrangement, including its ethology.

Admittedly, these speculations reach well beyond the data and require some liberalization of notions about discrimination, but the freedom to indulge in such lapses should be among the prerogatives of a discussant. A format such as this, however, does facilitate the mapping onto behavior theory of some of the phenomena of drug dependency and almost compulsive drug seeking that occur in the absence of true pharmacologic abstinence.

Dr. Goldberg (Chapter 4) has provided us with an elegant demonstration of the contribution of conditioning to drug taking and relapse by showing how some of the effects of nalorphine on morphine-dependent and post-dependent monkeys could be conditioned to a neutral stimulus with a Type-S procedure. It is important to note that only part of the "abstinence syndrome" evoked by nalorphine actually came under the control of the conditioned stimulus, and the responses that became conditioned did so at different rates. His demonstration of post-dependent sensitization to nalorphine should lead to a better understanding of physiologic mechanisms that contribute to the hardiness and persistence of drug seeking in post-dependent persons. Also, the data showed the specificity of this conditioning: the conditioned stimulus for nalorphine increased morphine self-injection but decreased lever pressing for food. It was not clear whether a conditioned emotional upset or whether conditioned gastric disturbance that interfered with hunger produced the conditioned suppression of food-seeking behavior, but the fact of the conditioning as such was clear and unambiguous. The precision of these techniques and the specificity of the results pave the way for extended critical analysis of conditioned components in morphine dependence and relapse.

Though abstinence, and conditioning with respect to it, certainly play important roles in dependence and relapse, dependency has other supports as well, relating to pleasures and rewards other than the relief of abstinence. Some are direct, such as the relief of pain, anxiety, and tension. Others are indirect and may involve the development of adventitious discriminations such as were suggested in connection with the conditioning of drug effects of activity. And these may occur in combination. The fat man, who must reduce, partially cuts himself off from the pleasant social rituals and fellowship associated with dining. Reformed cigarette smokers comment on their empty hands and unfilled motoric patterns, and reach for cigarettes long after their pharmacologic dependence on nicotine has disappeared. The light narcosis induced by a martini makes obligatory cocktail parties and business luncheons bearable, and in so doing favors differential reinforcement of drinking by commercial consummations and other stimuli quite removed from the direct effects of the alcohol. Drug taking and other dependencies thus may be supported partly in that they produce states or behaviors which confer preferential access to important rewards that are independent of the drug effect simply by making the behavior that leads to such rewards possible or more probable.

Drug abuse in the service of pleasure is hard to study at the animal level because animals usually become dependent only as we force it on them, or under rather special circumstances. For humans, the problem is ubiquitous and complex, and the pleasures involved are not always apparent to the nonaddicted eye. Some heroin users are less than enthusiastic about methadone treatment, even though that drug substitutes for heroin and relieves abstinence. Apparently, it deprives them of "highs," in which they get gratification in fantasy, and also removes them from the "excitements" of the "addict way of life." To us, these "highs," while the user is "on the nod," look uninspiring, and the "addict way of life" unattractive. Perhaps the heroin user really hesitates to relinquish his access to "time out" from a dull and nagging life, and his descriptions are a gloss. We do not know. The point is that functional analysis of dependent behavior rather than testimony will be required to clarify these problems; but in the development of the analysis we would be foolish indeed to disregard the hints that dependent persons give us as to what is important.

Becker's picture (1953) of how one learns to use marihuana for pleasure described the process from a sociologist's point of view, but his sequence (with a few rhetorical adjustments) is coordinate with factors that would loom large in a behavioral analysis. First, of course, there must exist some situation that conduces to trying the drug. Rebellion, imitation, curiosity, social pressures, and the like are required to raise the operant level enough so that the person actually smokes it several times. Then the person must learn how to identify the drug effect, how to smoke in such a way as to regulate or maximize the effect, and to connect it with drug use. Finally, he has to define this effect as good or pleasurable, even though initially he probably did not find it so. While withdrawal effects may be sufficient to mediate these transformations for narcotics, other contingencies probably govern this rediscrimination for drugs that are not associated with abstinence effects. The adventitious discriminations suggested earlier may be one type of contingency that participates; doubtless there are others. In any event, the use of drugs for pleasure must involve multiple steps in conditioning, with Type-S, Type-R, and discriminative control combined at all stages.[1]

REFERENCE

Becker, H.S. Becoming a marihuana user. *Amer. J. Sociol.*, 1953, 59, 235.

Unconditioned Stimulus Functions of Drugs: Interpretations. II

Milton A. Trapold

Department of Psychology
University of Minnesota
Minneapolis, Minnesota

I do not have the expertise to comment upon the relevance of the data presented in these chapters to our understanding of specific drug effects, so I will not even try.

Rather, what I would like to do is draw upon a possible parallel between studies using drugs as unconditioned stimuli and research on classical conditioning using food, shock, and other conventional reinforcing agents, that may suggest fruitful avenues for future drug-conditioning research.

Over the years, researchers who have worked on non-drug classical conditioning have slowly but consistently shifted their thinking about the significance of classical conditioning as a procedure for bringing about changes in behavior. Early, the emphasis was placed upon the fact that when you pair a conditioned stimulus (CS) with some unconditioned stimulus (US), the CS acquires the capacity to control some particular response, or at most a quite limited set of specific responses. However, given that view of classical conditioning, it is very difficult to use classical conditioning to explain very much behavior. The list of behaviors that can be transferred directly to new stimuli via classical conditioning is simply too short to gain much explanatory purchase on the total range of behaviors that a rat or dog or monkey, let alone a human, is capable of evidencing.

However, that fact has not resulted in the relegation of classical conditioning to the status of a laboratory curiosity, and the reason is that what gets conditioned to a CS by virtue of having been paired with a US is not just a limited set of specific responses. At least for such well-studied USs as food and electric shock, what appears to get conditioned is a state, which, over and above eliciting specific changes in cardiovascular activity, skin resistance, salivation, and the like, also possesses a number of properties that are important in the control of operant behavior. That is, the state of affairs that gets conditioned on the basis of a particular US can operate to control essentially any chunk of operantly learnable behavior, given the proper learning history and the proper circumstances for observing the control.

The most obvious example is the ability of some USs to imbue CSs with the capacity to function as reinforcers. Thus, a CS for food, quite apart from the fact that it may control conditioned responses like salivation or chewing movements, also can be used to strengthen or maintain operants upon which it is made contingent. Similarly, a CS for shock will reinforce behaviors contingent upon its offset.

Another well-known example of such a functional property is the one that Dr. Goldberg (Chapter 4) made use of in his studies of conditioning based upon nalorphine—namely, the ability of some CSs to suppress or facilitate a wide range of ongoing behaviors. Like nalorphine CSs, shock CSs suppress many responses but facilitate others, most notably avoidance responses. Similarly, a CS for food sometimes facilitates ongoing food-getting behavior, and sometimes interferes with ongoing avoidance responding.

Results such as these have led numerous theorists to propose that the state conditioned to a CS by virtue of pairings with food or shock possesses motivational properties of some kind (Rescorla and Solomon, 1967).

Recent research in our lab has shown that the state of affairs conditioned to a CS for food possesses stimulus properties that can gain stimulus control over operants reinforced in their presence. Moreover, we have shown that the stimulus properties of the state conditioned on the basis of one type of food US are different from that conditioned on the basis of another type of food; one operant can be brought under the control of the expectation of solid food, while concurrently a different one is brought under the control of the expectation of sugar water.

This is not the place for a detailed discussion of these and possibly other operant-controlling properties of the state that gets conditioned when you pair a CS with food or shock. Rather, I mention them merely to make the point that for these USs, at least, many researchers have come to the conclusion that the real significance of classical conditioning, the thing about it that is going to contribute most to our ability to predict and control behavior in general, is not the specific response-controlling properties of the CS, but the functional properties it acquires which give it the potential of controlling a wide range of operant behavior.

This conclusion has led some of us to adopt a research strategy that may

Unconditioned Stimulus Functions of Drugs: Interpretations 81

be applicable in the study of drug-based conditioning. This strategy plays down the measurement of specific conditioned responses, and concentrates on studying the operant-controlling aspects of the conditioned state. There are several reasons for adopting this strategy. First, of course, is the fact that operant-controlling effects are what we are primarily interested in. Second, and perhaps as important, is that while there is some covariation between the operant-controlling properties of the conditioned state and specific conditioned responses, this covariation is in general not good enough to let us make inferences about the operant-controlling effects from the specific conditioned responses. A very nice instance of this is Dr. Goldberg's finding that whereas all his monkeys showed nalorphine-based conditioned suppression of food-reinforced behavior, three of the five did not show concomitant conditioning of emesis, salivation, or heart rate, and none showed conditioned respiration or temperature changes.

Adopting this strategy means, in effect, that once you know something functions as a US, by showing conditioned changes in some specific response, you then cease any special interest in that specific response and begin to wonder about the more general operant-controlling properties of the state. In the work of Pickens and Dougherty (Chapter 3), for instance, this strategy would lead one to drop activity as a measure of conditioning, or at least as the only measure of conditioning, once it has been ascertained that amphetamines condition something, and go on to concentrate on such questions as: "Do CSs for amphetamine function as conditioned reinforcers?" "Does a CS for amphetamine facilitate when superimposed upon an amphetamine-reinforced baseline of behavior?" "What does it do when superimposed upon baselines maintained by other reinforcers?" "Can the amphetamine-conditioned state become a cue for a specific operant?" And so on.

In the case of Dr. Goldberg's work, the strategy leads me to wonder whether the nalorphine-conditioned state is aversive. Will it function as a negative reinforcer? If so, do these properties vary across morphine-naive, dependent, and post-dependent subjects? Can it be used as a punisher? It also leads me to wonder about the source of the differences in nalorphine-based conditioned suppression when the baseline behavior was morphine reinforced, as compared to when it was food reinforced. Is this similar to the differential effects of a shock CS on food and avoidance baselines? That is, is this a case where the operant-controlling properties of the conditioned state interact in some fundamental way with the source of reinforcement for the baseline behavior? We can't tell from Dr. Goldberg's data because the CS-nalorphine interval, nalorphine dose used as US, ambient morphine level, and baseline response rate all differed in the two cases. But it is an important question, and one that has received little attention in general. Just why do CSs sometimes facilitate and sometimes suppress ongoing behavior?

The basic question to be answered about any specific instance of classical conditioning, and about classical conditioning in general, is, "What gets learned?" The complete answer is not in yet for any instance of conditioning, but from those cases that have been studied most the partial answer to date is, a lot more than specific peripheral responses. Moreover, it is my opinion that the real importance of classical conditioning, whether it be based on shock or on drugs, lies in this "a lot more." If classically conditioned drug effects are to be of general behavioral significance, it seems to me beyond question that that significance will reside in their ability to push operant behavior around.

I am not familiar enough with the drug conditioning literature to know whether I am arguing for a position or strategy that is already generally accepted—I may be, inasmuch as Dr. Goldberg's work on nalorphine conditioning follows it closely. Since the point of view I have argued is still not explicitly articulated by very many traditional classical conditioning researchers, I thought it worthwhile to bring it up in this context.

Another point which devolves from research on the operant-controlling properties of CSs for food and shock is that stimuli that signal the active nonoccurrence of these events also seem to acquire active operant-controlling properties. In other words, under some circumstances, as yet poorly understood, nonoccurrence of a US itself acts as a US for a state that also has the power to push operants around. A CS for the nonoccurrence of food sometimes becomes a good negative reinforcer, and sometimes produces increases in responding when superimposed upon a completely independently established shock avoidance baseline. Similarly, a CS for nonoccurrence of shock sometimes acquires positive reinforcing properties, and inhibits when superimposed upon an ongoing baseline of avoidance responding.

Are there such "negative CS" effects in drug-based conditioning? What would be the effect of a CS for nonoccurrence of amphetamine upon independently established amphetamine-reinforced baseline behavior? On other types of behavioral baselines, both drug reinforced and conventionally reinforced? Would it function as a negative reinforcer? Similar questions could be asked about signals for the nonoccurrence of morphine or nalorphine, or any drug for that matter. I do not know what the answers will be, but whatever they are they cannot help but further our understanding not only of conditioned drug effects but also of the mechanism whereby the nonoccurrence of something becomes a US, and of the nature of what gets conditioned by virtue of the nonoccurrence of a US.

REFERENCES

Rescorla, R.A., and Solomon, R.L. Two-process learning theory: Relationships between Pavlovian conditioning and instrumental learning. *Psychol. Rev.*, 1967, 74, 151.

Trapold, M.A. Are expectancies based upon different positive reinforcing events discriminably different? *Learning and Motivation*, 1970, 1, 129-140.

SECTION 3

DISCRIMINATIVE STIMULUS FUNCTIONS OF DRUGS

Discriminative Control of Behavior by Drug States

Donald A. Overton

Eastern Pennsylvania Psychiatric Institute
Philadelphia, Pennsylvania

Centrally acting drugs can be used in place of discriminative stimuli, and often acquire response control with surprising rapidity when used in this way. Also, without discriminative training, the performance of behaviors learned while an animal is drugged may appear conditional upon the drug state present during response acquisition; the response may fail to transfer, or transfer only partially, into different drug states.

We are accustomed to the fact that the brain can store a variety of learned responses, and that only one of these may be performed on a particular occasion. A relatively trivial sensory event may determine which response occurs. Such discriminative control utilizes elaborate neural mechanisms for the detection and interpretation of sensory events. Response selection may also depend on naturally occurring internal states such as hunger, rage, and fatigue. We usually assume that specific neural systems detect, or generate, such internal states, and that these systems are interconnected with the rest of the brain in a manner which produces behavior appropriate to the internal state.

However, when arbitrarily selected drug states determine response selection, the situation looks less reasonable. The brain contains synapses sensitive to drugs which we might call receptors, but no system is known that collects or integrates information about the drug state of the animal. There is no obvious adaptive value to organizing the brain so that response selection can be contingent upon such nonphysiological internal states. Also, because the drug states are not necessarily similar to naturally occurring physiological states, there has been no evolutionary opportunity to develop mechanisms to mediate such response control. Nonetheless, drugs can acquire discriminative control of behavior, and we are led to ask how they do so.

Two general types of proposals are usually advanced to account for discriminative control by drug states. One type of hypothesis holds that the drugs are somehow tapping in on and utilizing the systems that primarily developed to allow sensory control of behavior. Such a hypothesis is parsimonious in that it only postulates CNS properties which are already well demonstrated, i.e., the mechanisms which mediate discriminative control by sensory stimuli. The title of this book, *Stimulus Properties of Drugs*, tends to focus attention on this possible mechanism.

A second type of hypothesis holds that response selection by drug states illustrates some intrinsic property of the brain, and that the sensory systems are not involved. It follows that the characteristics of discriminative control by drug states must be determined by properties of the brain rather than by properties of the sensory systems. One version of this second hypothesis holds that response selection by drug states demonstrates in exaggerated form the operation of mechanisms that are also involved in the control by behavior by naturally occurring internal states. Another version postulates that response control by drugs involves processes that are not involved in the control of behavior under natural conditions.

This chapter will review evidence bearing on the question of whether response selection by drug states utilizes the usual mechanisms for sensory control, or whether some other central mechanism is involved. We will first review experiments that illustrate the effectiveness of drugs as discriminative or conditional stimuli. These data define some characteristics of the phenomenon to be explained, and somewhat restrict the range of possible mechanisms to which we can attribute the stimulus properties of drugs. Then we will examine in more detail data concerned with the question of whether drugs actually produce distinguishable stimuli.

PROCEDURES

Most of the data presented in this chapter have been obtained with a T-maze in which rats are trained to escape from shock. On each trial the rat is dropped into the start box of the maze with the shock already turned on and is allowed to run freely in the maze until it reaches the correct goal box where the grid floor is unshocked. Ten such trials are administered each day in a single 10-minute training session. Drugs are administered prior to the training session, and training occurs during the period of maximal apparent drug effect. Typically, the rat is required to discriminate between two drug states. On successive days the imposed drug state alternates, as does the required choice. Hence, a right turn is always required under one drug state and a left turn under the second drug state.

The T-maze is an easy task, and rats can learn to run to the left (or right) goal box in a few trials. If the selected drug states are indistinguishable, the drug discrimination task amount to repeated reversal training. Each day the rats are required to run in a direction opposite to that required on the previous day. They typically make an incorrect choice on the first trial, thus performing the response learned on the previous day, and thereafter make correct responses on trials 2 to 10. If the imposed drug states are distinguishable, rats learn after a few sessions to perform the correct response even on the first trial of each daily training session. In this case, the first trial choice is determined by the imposed drug state and is opposite to the responses made during the preceeding session.

EFFECTIVE CNS DRUGS

Figure 1 shows learning curves as differential responding developed in four groups of rats required to differentiate four different doses of pentobarbital from the nondrug condition. All doses except 5 mg/kg were differentiated from the nondrug state within 16 sessions, and high doses

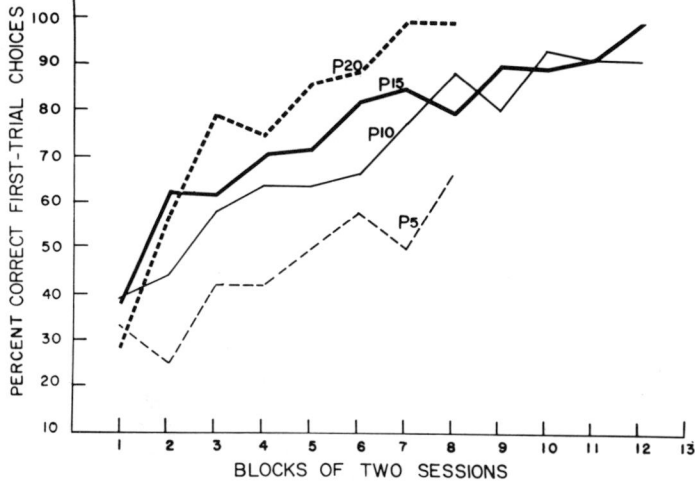

Fig. 1. Learning curves for rats required to differentiate various doses of pentobarbital from the no-drug condition. X-axis: Successive blocks of two training sessions each. Y-axis: Percentage of first trial choices that were correct. Labels indicate dose in mg/kg. $N \geq 6$ per group.

allowed response control to develop more rapidly than low doses (p < .01). Apparently the high doses were in some sense more "distinctive," although it is not clear whether the rats "perceived" the drug state. Several other anesthetic drugs have been tested. All produce a state that can be readily differentiated from the nondrug condition, and the states produced by these drugs are apparently indistinguishable from one another if dosages are suitably adjusted (Overton, 1966). For each of these anesthetic drugs the dose required to produce a noticeable ataxia is the minimal dose that can be easily differentiated from no drug. Also, the distinctive actions of pentobarbital can be reversed by the convulsant drug bemegride, just as are the anesthetic effects of pentobarbital. It does not follow that ataxia *causes* the drug state distinctiveness. However, it does appear that the drug actions which allow anesthetics to control T-maze choice are probably the same actions that produce their more familiar hypnotic and anesthetic effects.

In order to compare the distinctiveness of various pairs of drug conditions, it is convenient to record the number of training sessions before each rat reaches a criterion level of performance. For example, performance of the various groups in Figure 1 is shown by one line (Na Pentobarbital) in Figure 2. At the low-dose end of this dose-response curve, rats were trained a maximum of 60 sessions; if a rat had not achieved criterion performance by that time, a score of 60 was assigned for the performance of that rat. Referring to the figure, we can see that pentobarbital doses lower than 5

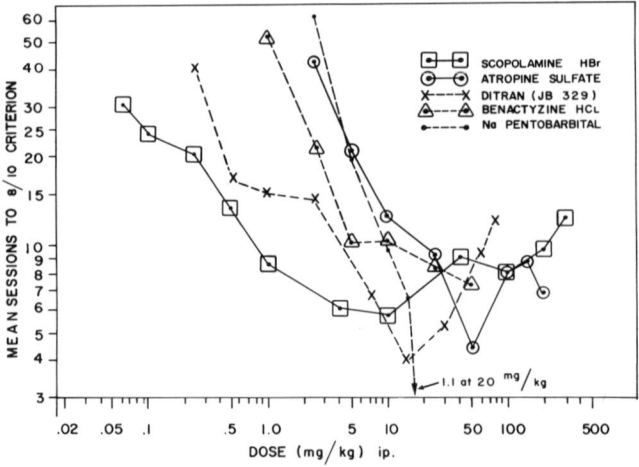

Fig. 2. Dose response curves for antimuscarinic drugs and for pentobarbital. X-axis: Intraperitoneal dose. Y-axis: Mean number of sessions before the beginning of criterion performance (8 correct first-trial choices in 10 successive training sessions) by rats trained to differentiate drug from no drug. N≥3 per data point.

mg/kg were not differentiated from no drug within 60 sessions, and that increasing doses were differentiated from the no-drug condition with increasing rapidity (up to 25 mg/kg, beyond which anesthesia results).

Antimuscarinic drugs constitute a second group of easily distinguishable drugs. The relevant actions of the antimuscarinic drugs are apparently different from those of the anesthetic drugs, because rats can easily distinguish between antimuscarinic and anesthetic drug states (Overton, 1966). Figure 2 shows dose-response curves for four antimuscarinic drugs indicating the rapidity with which each dose was differentiated from the no-drug condition. For low doses of each drug, the negative slope of the dose response curve is similar to that observed with pentobarbital. However as dosage increases, the distinctiveness of the antimuscarinic drugs appears asymptotic; antimuscarinic drugs never achieve at any dosage a distinctiveness much greater than that shown by pentobarbital 15 mg/kg. A similar plateau of activity has been observed in other experiments on the neurochemical and behavioral effects of high doses of atropine and scopolamine (Giarman and Pepeu, 1964; White, Nash, Westerbeke, and Possanza, 1961). An apparent decrease in distinctiveness is observed with very high doses of antimuscarinic drugs, but this is probably an artefact. It seems unlikely that the drugs become less distinctive as dosage is raised. Instead the required training probably increases with very high doses because of generally impaired maze learning ability.

Nicotine and related nicotinic drugs constitute a third group of easily distinguishable agents. Nicotinic drugs can be distinguished from anesthetics, antimuscarinics, and from the nicotinic blocking agent, mecamylamine. Mecamylamine itself can be distinguished from the nondrug state, and this antinicotinic drug strongly antagonizes the "distinctive" effects of nictoine (Overton, 1969).

Table 1 lists all the centrally acting drugs that have been tested for discriminative control up to the present time. Most distinctive drugs are in one of nine pharmacologic groups. In addition, several other active and inactive drugs are listed. Most of the data supporting this table have been collected in T-maze experiments similar to those described above (Overton, 1968b, 1969). Some drugs are rather tentatively included, inasmuch as they have not been extensively studied.

The available data indicate that drugs with similar pharmacologic actions are relatively indistinguishable from each other when equally effective doses are compared. However, drugs in each of the listed categories can be distinguished rather easily from those in each of the other categories, except that anesthetics and minor tranquilizers can perhaps not be distinguished. Surprisingly, certain drugs (e.g., Dilantin) are barely distinguishable from no

Table 1. *Centrally acting drugs tested for discriminative control*

STRONG CONTROL	MODERATE	WEAK
Anesthetics	**Antimuscarinic Drugs**	**Phenothiazines**
Pentobarbital 10-20	Atropine 20-200	Chlorpromazine 4
Phenobarbital 60-80	Scopolamine 1-300	Acepromazine 8
Secobarbital 15-20	Benactyzine 10-50	Perphenazine 5
Na Barbital 150	Ditran 5-60	Prothipendyl 12
Amobarbital 30	**Nicotinic Drugs**	**Dibenzazepines**
Chloral Hydrate 150	Nicotine 1-4	Imipramine 20
Ethyl Alcohol 1000-3000	Lobeline 40	**Relatively Inactive Drugs**
Paraldehyde 300	Antagonist: Mecamylamine	Pryilamine 50
Progesterone 125	**Narcotics**	Phenoxybenzamine 10
Hydroxydione 25	Morphine 9-36	Physostigmine 1
Ethyl Carbamate	**Antinicotinic Drugs**	Dilantin 175
Ether	Mecamylamine 10-30	
Nitrous Oxide	**Convulsants**	
Antagonist: Bemegride	Metrazol 30	
Minor Tranquilizers	Bemegride 7.5	
Librium 30	**Other Drugs**	
Meprobamate 200	Amphetamine 1-5	
	Mescaline 50	
	Acetylcholine (In dogs)	
	Epinephrine (In dogs)	
	Norepinephrine (In dogs)	
	Erythroidine (In dogs	

NOTE: Tested dose levels are given beside each drug in mg/kg for i.p. injection in the rat. The ordering according to relative effectiveness is only approximate and refers to the maximally effective tested dose of each drug. References can be found in Overton, 1968b.

drug even though these drugs have substantial CNS effects. In man, drug abuse rarely involves the drugs in Column 3 of Table 1, and this may be related to their relatively insignificant stimulus properties.

The multiplicity of distinguishable drug states discourages many interpretations of this phenomenon, and points to the need for rather differentiated models to explain how drugs achieve response control. For example, one apparently inadequate model postulates that the drugs induce shifts along naturally occurring internal continua (e.g., arousal, hunger, thirst) which in turn acquire response control. This explanation becomes increasingly untenable as the dimensionality of the internal "drug space" increases, because there appear to be more distinguishable drug states than internal mediators. Also, hunger and thirst do not acquire response control in the T-maze nearly as rapidly as do many of the more effective drugs listed in Table 1, and thus one cannot easily argue that variations in these drive levels mediate response control by drugs (Overton, 1964).

DISCRIMINATIVE CONTROL IN VARIOUS TASKS

Drugs can acquire discriminative control of behavior in a variety of tasks, as shown in Table 2. Most of these studies used saline and one of the

Table 2. Tasks in which drugs have controlled differential responding

Task	Required Responses State 1	Required Responses State 2	Motivation	Reference
T-Maze	Right	Left	Escape Shock	Overton (1964)
T-Maze	Black	White	Avoid Shock	Bindra and Reichert (1966)
T-Maze	Buzzer-Right No Buzzer-Left	Buzzer-Left No Buzzer-Right	Escape Shock	Phillips (1967)
Y-Maze	Right	Left	Food	Barry, Koepfer, and Lutch (1965)
3-Compartment Box	Right	Left	Escape Shock	Stewart (1962)
3-Alley Maze	3 States &	3 Responses	Escape Shock	Overton (1967)
Jumping Stand	Black Door	White Door	Food & Shock	Brown, Feldman, and Moore (1968)
Telescope Alley	Approach	Avoid	Food & Shock	Conger (1951)
Shuttlebox	Go	No-Go	Avoid Shock	Holmgren (1964)
Bar Press	Right Bar	Left Bar	Food	Kubena and Barry (1969); Harris and Balster (1970)
Bar Press	S_D=Light On	S_D=Light Off	Avoid Shock	Barry (1968)
Bar Press	FR-50	DRL-20	Food	Harris and Balster (1968, 1970)
Bar Press	Bar Press	No Response	Approach/Avoid	Kubena and Barry (1969)
Bar Press-Monkeys	Bar Press	No Response	Food	Schuster and Brady (1970)
Color Disc-Monkeys	S+=Color 1	S+=Color 2	Food	Bliss, Sledjeski and Leiman (1970)
Leg Flexion-Dogs	Right Leg	Left Leg	Avoid Shock	Girden and Culler (1937)
Leg Flexion-Dogs	Leg Flexion CR	No Response	Avoid Shock	Cook, Davidson, Davis and Kelleher (1960)

anesthetic drugs as the discriminative conditions, and differential responding typically appeared rather rapidly.

Although the nature of the stimulus is unclear, other characteristics of the acquisition of discriminative control by drug states appear to be similar to those of the discrimination learning that occurs when sensory stimuli are used. In the T-maze, for example, vicarious trial-and-error behavior is often observed at the choice point. The investigators listed in Table 2 are unanimous in failing to report any unusual behavior during the acquisition of drug-state discriminations. The absence of such reports suggests that behavior during the acquisition of drug-state discriminations is similar to that seen when sensory discriminations are formed in all these tasks, except that the stimulus is invisible to the investigator.

In addition to indicating that drugs are effective as stimuli in a variety of tasks, the table suggests that the phylogenetic range of the phenomenon is wide, inasmuch as rats, dogs, and monkeys have all shown differential responses controlled by drug state. However, as there are no reported failures to obtain response control with drugs, the table simply reflects tasks in which investigators have so far attempted to establish response control with drug states. It does not allow us to delimit the range of tasks or species in which this phenomenon will occur.

DRUGS AND STIMULI: FORMAL SIMILARITIES

State-dependent learning resembles stimulus generalization. Without explicit discriminative training, a response learned in one drug state may fail to appear after the drug condition has been changed. Most experiments have utilized the nondrug condition and one drug state, thus testing only one point on the generalization gradient. Gradients for transfer to a variety of doses have usually not been established. In the T-maze task virtually no transfer of training is observed between the drug condition produced by 25 mg/kg pentobarbital and the nondrug condition (Overton, 1964). However, with lower doses transfer becomes more complete (Bindra and Reichert, 1967; Overton, 1968b).

Table 3 lists the tasks in which state-dependent (dissociated) learning has been investigated. Dissociation can be produced by much lower doses in some of these tasks than in others. This suggests that steeper generalization gradients are observed in some tasks than in others. Several of the experiments in Table 3 have yielded results indicating that learning which took place in the drug condition failed to transfer into the nondrug condition, whereas learning which occurred in the no-drug condition transferred without decrement to the drug condition (Barnhart, 1967; Overton, 1968b). Asymmetrical transfer between two different drug states has also been observed (Berger and Stein, 1969b). It is not clear whether such asymmetrical dissociation is a bona fide phenomenon; it may represent the summation of a symmetrical generalization decrement with some other drug effect (Berger and Stein, 1969a). However, taken at face value, asymmetrical dissociation does not directly parallel the findings of most stimulus generalization experiments.

Acquired discriminative control of learned responses by drug states is a second phenomenon which leads us to say that drugs have stimulus properties. The results suggest that the drug states produced by each class of drugs in Table 1 constitute the basis for something equivalent to a sensory continuum, with various doses of each drug producing different points along the continuum. Rats can differentiate between drug conditions on the different continua (which are produced by drugs in the different classes). Along a given continuum, high (intense) doses may be differentiated from saline more rapidly than low doses, and rats may differentiate between a high and a low dose of a single drug (Overton, 1968a). Considered from this

Table 3. Tasks in which dissociated learning has been studied

Tasks	Anesthetics	Anticholinergics	Narcotics	Phenothiazines	Curare	Amphetamines	Investigators
Straight Alley–Food	+–						Barry, Wagner, and Miller (1962); Iwahara, Nagamura, and Iwasaki (1967)
T-Maze–Position	+–	+					Bindra and Reichert (1967); Carlson (1967); Hill, Jones and Bell (1970); Overton (1964); Ross (1967); Seymore (1967)
Black/White Maze Disc	+–						Bindra and Reichert (1966); Caul (1967)
Temporal Maze–Food	+						Chen (1968)
Telescope Alley	+–						Barry, Miller, and Tidd (1962); Conger (1951); Grossman and Miller
Hole-in-wall Escape		+					Paskal (1962)
One-Way CAR	+	+–	–				Bindra, Nyman, and Wise (1965); Bindra and Reichert (1966); Burgoyne (1968); Daley (1968); Doty and Doty (1963)
Shuttlebox CAR	+–	+–				+	Ader and Clink (1957); Barnhart and Abbott (1967); Crow (1966); Holmgren (1964, 1965); Kamano and Arp (1964); Leiman, Bliss, Powers and Rosenzweig (1967); Oliverio (1968); Sachs, Weingarten, and Klein (1966); Shmavonian (1956)
Pole-Climb CAR		+		+			Gruber, Stone, and Reed (1967); Otis (1964)
Pit-Escape CAR				+		+	Lal (1969)
Step-Down Avoidance	–						Calhoun and Smith (1968); Meyers (1965)
Dark-Hole Avoidance	–	–				–	Bohdanecky and Jarvik (1967); Iwahara, Iwasaki, and Hasegawa (1968); Stark (1967)
Bar Press	–	–	+	–		+	Belleville (1964); Charney and Reynolds (1967); Crow (1970); Harris and Balster (1970)
Conditioned Freezing	+						Bindra, Nyman, and Wise (1965)
Conditioned Anorexia	+–	+–					Berger and Stein (1969a; 1969b); Evans and Patton (1968); Paskal (1962); Tenen (1967); Vogel, Hughes, and Carlton (1967)
CER (Suppressed Bar Press)	+–			+–			Barry, Etheredge, and Miller (1965); Cicala and Hartley (1967); Heistad (1957, 1958); Heistad and Torres (1959); Kanzler (1967); Sherman (1967)
Habituation to Novelty	+–	+				–	Bindra and Reichert (1967); Carlton and Vogel (1965); Marriott and Spencer (1965); Oliverio (1968); Rushton, Steinberg, and Tinson (1963); Shillito (1967)
Y-Maze–Goldfish	+						Ryback (1969)
Imprinting–Checks	–						Bradford and Macdonald (1969)
Cond. Leg Flexion–Dog					+–		Cook, Davidson, Davis, and Kelleher (1960); Gardner and McCollough (1962); Girden (1940); Girden and Culler (1937); Solomon (1962)

Note: + indicates a report of dissociation
— indicates a report with dissociation not observed

Table 3. (cont.)

Tasks	Anesthetics	Anticholinergics	Narcotics	Phenothiazines	Curare	Amphetamines	Investigators
Color Disc–Monkeys	+						Bliss, Sledjeski, and Leiman (1970)
Visual Learning–Man	+–			–		+	Bustamante, Jordan, Vila, Gonzalez, and Insua (1970); Goodwin, Powell, Bremer, Haine, and Stern (1969); Kurland, Cassel, and Goldberg (1968); Osborn, Bunker, Cooper, Frank, and Hilgard (1967)
Verbal Learning–Man	+–					+	Bustamante, Rossello, Jordan, Pradere, and Insua (1968); Caird (1968); Goodwin, Powell, Bremer, Haine, and Stern (1969); Madill (1967); Osborn, Bunker, Cooper, Frank, and Hilgard (1967); Storm and Caird (1967); Tarter (1968)
Operant Learning–Man	+						Goodwin, Powell, Bremer, Haine, and Stern (1969); Madill (1967)
Motor Skill–Man	+–						Caird (1968); Madill (1967)

Note: + indicates a report of dissociation
      – indicates a report with dissociation not observed

perspective the nondrug state becomes only a particular point in a multidimensional "drug space"—the point of intersection of the several continua that may be generated by various doses of each of the effective drugs.

The two phenomena, drug-state discrimination and dissociation, appear to reflect the different training procedures used to generate the results, but do not indicate to this author that different properties of drugs are responsible for the two effects. As with sensory discriminations, response control may be acquired by two drug conditions which are sufficiently similar so that no substantial generalization decrement would be produced by state change in the absence of prior discriminative training. Thus the discriminative training procedure is a more sensitive test for the stimulus properties of drugs than is a dissociation (2 × 2) procedure. In the T-maze, as one requires rats to discriminate increasingly high doses of pentobarbital from the nondrug state, acquisition of response control becomes increasingly rapid. If a discriminative training procedure is used with pentobarbital 25 mg/kg, the data appear as discriminative learning curves. However, differential responding appears as soon as the rat can learn the response that is required in each drug state, and apparently does not involve much sharpening of the pretraining generalization gradient. The results suggest that little transfer of training between the drug and no-drug conditions takes place, and this can be directly demonstrated with slightly different training procedures (Overton, 1964; Seymore, 1967).

Although drug-state discrimination and dissociation in the T-maze appear to reflect the same properties of drugs, it is not certain that all the reports of state-dependent learning listed in Table 3 reflect these same drug effects. Leaving aside the issue of whether all of these findings can be replicated, the differences in required dose level and the frequent observation of asymmetrical dissociation suggest that other drug effects may be responsible for some of these results. Much more work will be required to adequately demonstrate that the positive reports in Table 3 reflect a single phenomenon and not simply a melange of various drug effects.

One recent experiment in our laboratories suggests that a learning set develops during the acquisition of a drug-state discrimination, such that subsequent discriminations in the T-maze are more easily learned. Specifically, seven rats were first trained to discriminate alcohol 2,000 mg/kg from no drug, and after criterion performance was reached they were retrained with a right turn required when the maze was illuminated and a left turn required when the maze was totally dark. The light/dark training was a series of single trials spaced 15 minutes apart with the light/dark condition alternating on successive trials. For some rats the correct choice when the maze was dark corresponded to the previous alcohol choice; for other rats, the correct dark choice corresponded to the previous no-drug choice. These rats required a mean of 10.7 trials to begin criterion performance (9 out of 10 successive correct choices) of the light/dark discrimination. A control group without prior alcohol versus no-drug discrimination training required a mean of 31.6 trials to reach the same criterion on the light/dark discrimination task. This result is statistically significant ($p < .05$, t test) but is not conclusive for various reasons, such as the unequal age of the two groups at the time of light/dark training. Perhaps discriminative control by a pair of drug states would also appear more rapidly in rats that had previously been trained with a different pair of drug states. Such a demonstration of learning set would add to the list of similarities between stimulus and drug-state discrimination learning.

PERIPHERALLY ACTING DRUGS

One hypothetical mechanism by which centrally acting drugs might acquire discriminative control is by the production of proprioceptive or autonomic stimuli that rats can discriminate. This model predicts that drug-state and stimulus discriminations will have similar characteristics because rats trained with distinguishable drug states will actually be discriminating between sensory stimuli induced by the drugs. The following experiments bear directly on this hypothesis.

Antimuscarinic drugs are available in both quaternary and tertiary forms. With some degree of error we can say that the quaternary and tertiary antimuscarinics produce the same peripheral actions, and do so at equal doses, whereas tertiary antimuscarinic drugs are usually found to be at least 10 times more effective than quaternary forms in producing CNS actions (Longo, 1966). In this experiment two groups of rats were trained. One group differentiated atropine 25 mg/kg from no drug, and the second group differentiated atropine methyl nitrate 40 mg/kg from no drug. Rats trained with atropine began criterion performance after a mean of 9.5 training sessions, whereas rats trained with atropine methyl nitrate required 41 training sessions. Referring to Figure 2 we can see that atropine methyl nitrate 40 mg/kg was about as distinctive as atropine 2.5 mg/kg. The relative potency of these two drugs indicates that their peripheral actions were not responsible for discriminative control.

One obvious effect of pentobarbital is motor ataxia. Overton (1964) tested whether response selection could be based on proprioceptive cues resulting from muscle flaccidity induced by gallamine, a curare-like drug. Gallamine is a difficult drug to use for this purpose as the lethal dose is only slightly higher than the dose adequate to produce moderate ataxia. On the basis of preliminary screening, six rats were selected in which gallamine 7.5 mg/kg produced a noticeable but nonlethal muscle flaccidity. These rats were trained to discriminate gallamine 7.5 mg/kg from no drug. Figure 3 compares the performance of these animals with that of two other groups trained to differentiate pentobarbital 10 and 20 mg/kg, respectively, from no drug. During 50 sessions of training most gallamine rats approached (and one achieved) criterion performance at some point, but response control deteriorated subsequently in all cases. Since directly induced muscle flaccidity was relatively ineffective as a discriminative condition, we can conclude that response control by pentobarbital is probably not mediated to a substantial degree by drug-induced ataxia.

Table 4 lists several peripherally acting drugs that have been tested for their ability to acquire response control. Each of these drugs produces characteristically different and definable peripheral actions, which probably result in altered interoceptive stimuli, yet none provided an adequate basis for rapidly acquired discriminative control. No rats showed criterion performance within the indicated period of training, with the exception of one rat in the gallamine group and two in the methyl atropine group, as described

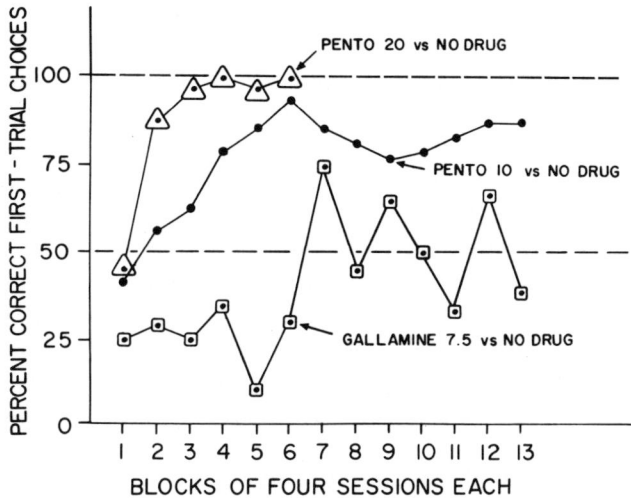

Fig. 3. Learning curves for rats required to differentiate gallamine or pentobarbital from no drug. X-axis: Blocks of four sessions each. Y-axis: Percentage of first-trial choices that were correct. N≥6 per group.

Table 4. *Peripherally acting drugs which have not rapidly acquired response-control*

Drug	Action	Number of Sessions of Training
Gallamine 7.5 mg/kg	Neuromuscular Blockade	50
Atropine Methyl Nitrate 40 mg/kg	Postganglionic Parasympathetic Blockade	50
Tetraethylammonium Chloride 40 mg/kg	Antinicotinic Ganglionic Blockade	40
Phenoxybenzamine 10 mg/kg	Alpha-Adrenergic Blockade	50
Adrenocorticotropic Hormone 5 units/kg	Adrenocorticosteroid Release	30

above. The conclusion appears justified that peripherally acting drugs are not nearly as distinguishable as are many centrally acting drugs. This finding opposes any hypothesis that postulates that CNS-active drugs achieve response control by inducing interoceptive stimuli.

RELATIVE EFFECTIVENESS OF DRUGS AND STIMULI

Drugs can acquire response control rapidly. Not only do drugs have discriminable effects but one sometimes gets the impression that their stimulus properties are more potent than those of "real" sensory stimuli.

This section will review some experiments that directly compare the control of learned responses by drugs and by interoceptive stimuli.

In an early experiment of this type (Overton, 1964), a discriminative stimulus "cocktail" consisting of differences on three sensory modalities was used. Specifically, six rats were required to turn right in the presence of a loud intermittent tone, a 2-ma shock level, and a bright light placed over the choice point. A left turn was required when the tone was eliminated, the shock reduced to 0.6 ma, and the room lights turned off (although some light was allowed to enter the room through an open door so that the maze was not totally dark). With these discriminative conditions, the rats reached criterion performance almost as rapidly as with pentobarbital 10 mg/kg. This demonstration that sensory stimuli can acquire control of response selection is hardly a unique finding. Our present interest centers about whether one of the sensory modalities used in this experiment may mediate response control by drug states.

The first candidate for investigation was shock level. Perhaps pentobarbital acquires response control by virtue of an analgesic effect which modulates shock-induced pain to a degree that rats can discriminate. Rats can hardly avoid "attending" to shock and it could be considered a "relevant" stimulus which might provide an adequate basis for response control.

Figure 4 shows learning curves obtained in two experiments in which differential shock conditions were used to establish control of T-maze

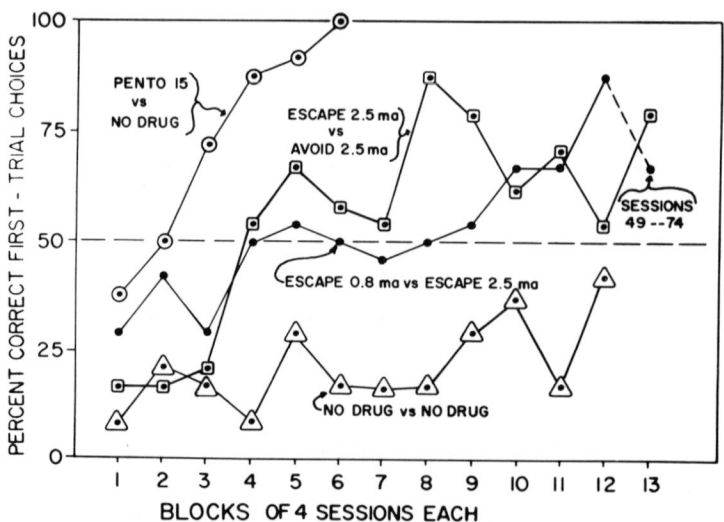

Fig. 4. The two middle learning curves are from groups required to select their T-maze choice on the basis of intensity of foot shock. N≥6 per group.

choice. Learning curves for a control group (ND versus ND) and for a phentobarbital versus no-drug group are also shown. One of the experimental groups was required to turn right during training sessions when the shock level was set to 0.8 ma and to turn left when the shock level was 2.5 ma (Grason-Stadler shock scrambler, Model E1064GS). In the second experimental group, right turns were required during sessions when the shock level was 2.5 ma. Left turns were required during alternate sessions (called avoidance sessions) during which the 2.5 ma shock was turned off when the rat was dropped into the maze and was only turned on 20 seconds later. During early avoidance training sessions, rats typically did not reach the correct goal box within 20 seconds and were thus shocked. However, subsequent to Session 15, the rats typically did avoid shock even on the first trial of avoidance sessions so that the task became one of turning right when shock was present and left when there was no shock. This avoid-left versus escape-right group made correct first trial choices much more often during avoidance sessions than during escape sessions. (The learning curve for Sessions 28 to 52 reflects nearly perfect performance during avoidance sessions and approximately 50 percent correct choices during escape sessions.) Such a large difference between performance under the two discriminative conditions is not usually seen when rats are trained to differentiate drug conditions, although performance during drug sessions is usually somewhat poorer than during nondrug sessions.

In both experimental groups, criterion performance began after an average of 28 sessions. Contrary to expectation, differential shock conditions did not rapidly acquire response control in the T-maze. This does not encourage us to believe that pentobarbital acquires response control via an analgesic action. Other experiments confirm the conclusion that drug-induced variations in the rats' sensitivity to shock do not to a substantial degree mediate discriminative control by pentobarbital in this task (Overton, 1968a).

Returning to the stimulus "cocktail" experiment (Overton, 1964), we see that we have followed a blind alley. That experiment suggested that differential shock conditions might rapidly acquire good discriminative control, and that such a discrimination might provide the basis for discriminative control by drug states. Neither of these possibilities turns out to be the case. Another possibility suggested by the stimulus "cocktail" experiment was that differential conditions of illumination might readily acquire response control in the T-maze.

Figure 5 shows learning curves for rats required to discriminate differing conditions of illumination. Rats in the group with the lowest learning curve were required to turn right when a 100-watt light bulb was placed 24 inches above the choice point and to turn left when a 7-watt bulb was placed above

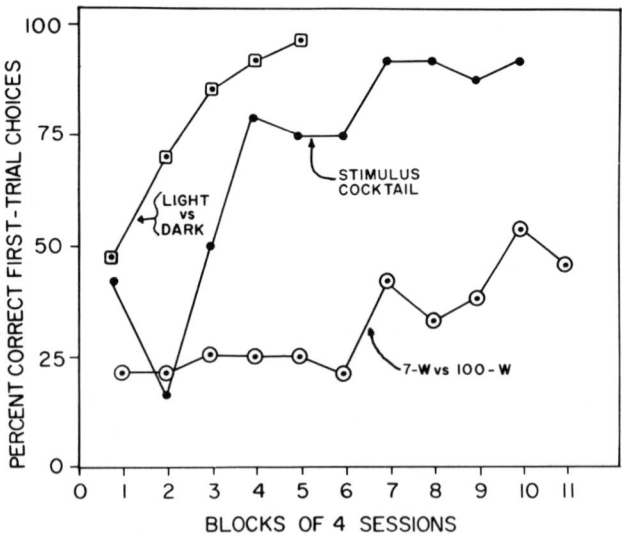

Fig. 5. Learning curves. The upper curve shows performance of a group required to turn right when the maze was lighted and left when it was totally dark. Conditions for the other groups are described in the text. N≥6 per group.

the choice point. Although these conditions were clearly discriminable to the investigator, they did not provide the rats with an adequate basis for discriminative control (no rats reached 8 to 10 criterion within 45 sessions). The middle learning curve was obtained in the stimulus "cocktail" experiment described above in which the illumination conditions were more distinguishable, and discriminative tone and shock conditions were also provided (mean sessions to begin criterion performance = 13). The figure shows that response control appeared most rapidly in the third group in which the rats were required to turn right when a 150-watt light bulb was placed above the choice point and to turn left when they were trained in *total* darkness. This group of rats required an average of five training sessions to reach the beginning of criterion performance, as do rats required to differentiate pentobarbital 15 mg/kg from no drug. In *some* rats response control appeared so rapidly as to suggest that a substantial generalization decrement occurred when illumination conditions were so drastically changed. Although response loss was not total, discriminative control in these cases appeared to be based on a partial inability to generalize between the two illumination conditions as much as on an acquired discrimination.

Moffett and Ettlinger (1967) reported a partial dissociation in monkeys between learning that took place in the light and in the dark. The possibility

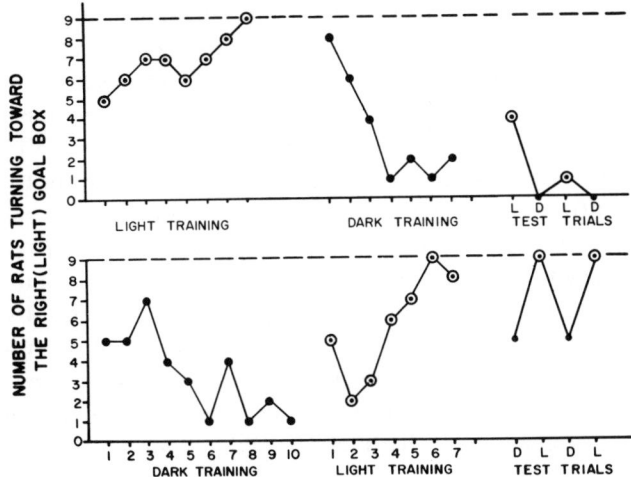

Fig. 6. Test for dissociation of responses learned in a lighted maze and in a totally darkened maze. Test trial performance does not indicate dissociation inasmuch as rats generally performed the most recently acquired response irrespective of the test trial illumination condition. N=9 per group.

of total dissociation has been investigated in the T-maze. Figure 6 shows the results. Individual training trials in this experiment were spaced 24 hours apart. The top half of the figure shows data for nine rats that received eight training trials to the right goal box with the maze lighted, followed by eight trials in the dark with a left turn required. After training, test trials were administered under both the light and dark conditions. During these test trials, both goal boxes were accessible. Two features of the data clearly indicate transfer of training between the light and dark conditions. On the first trial of reversal training, choices were predominantly toward the goal box that had been correct during the first block of training trials, indicating that this response was retained under the new conditions of illumination. Furthermore, during test trials the rats predominantly performed the response learned during the second block of training trials, independent of the conditions of illumination. The initially acquired response showed only a slight tendency to reappear under the original illumination condition, and even this trend is unconvincing as the number of light choices never exceeded 50 percent. The bottom half of the figure shows similar results obtained when the initial block of trials was performed under the dark condition. Similar results have also been obtained with two other groups where trials were spaced 15 minutes apart instead of 24 hours. The failure to find total dissociation is altogether as expected, because in the T-maze obvious transfer of training occurs between drug conditions that are only as discriminable as light and dark—e.g., pentobarbital 15 mg/kg and no drug.

It is worth emphasizing that among the variety of peripherally acting drugs and sensory stimuli discussed in this chapter, the conditions of light versus dark are the only conditions that acquired response control as rapidly as do many differential drug conditions. This encourages us to speculate that drugs may acquire discriminative control by producing changes in visual perception, which the rats then utilize as discriminative stimuli. However, available evidence does not support this hypothesis. Specifically, if sighted rats initially acquire a drug/no-drug discrimination and are then blinded, they continue to show T-maze choices appropriate to their current drug state after enucleation. Also, if rats are blinded before training, and are then trained to discriminate pentobarbital 15 mg/kg from no drug, their learning curve is only slightly below that that would be shown by sighted rats trained with the same drug conditions (Figure 7). Since drug-state discrimination is not abolished by a total interruption of visual input, it appears that this discrimination is not primarily based on modified perception of the visual world in normally sighted rats (Overton, 1968a.) The possibility remains that drugs might "produce" a visual stimulus (a sort of hallucination) by some

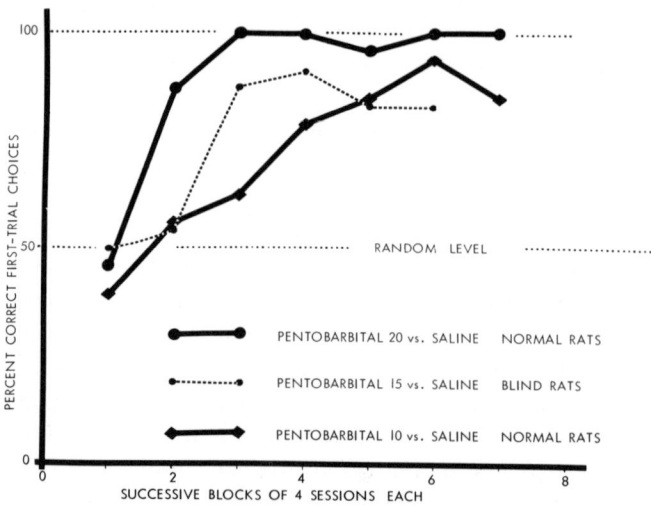

Fig. 7. Learning curves. The performance of a blind group of rats trained to differentiate pentobarbital 15 mg/kg from saline is compared with that of two groups of sighted rats also trained to differentiate pentobarbital from saline. N≥6 per group.

action on the visual system within the CNS, and that this stimulus might remain in enucleated rats.

Let us consider a hypothetical mechanism that might account for the stimulus properties of drugs. Perhaps drugs achieve response control by substantially impairing sensory perception in one or more modalities. Such a disorganization of sensory perception might have effects similar to those of deleting a sensory modality, e.g., by turning off the lights. The proposal is not that drugs achieve response control by producing discriminable stimuli in the usual sense, but that they act via disorganization of the mechanisms for sensory perception. The light versus dark experiments show that elimination of visual input does produce something like a partially dissociated state, in that rats deprived of visual input can rapidly learn a response opposite to that performed when vision is present. Although drug discriminations do not appear to be mediated by disruption of perception in the visual modality, similar generalization decrements might be produced by drug-induced disruption of other modalities. The first step in testing such a hypothesis would be to demonstrate that temporary disruption of other sensory modalities would allow a partial dissociation (rapid discrimination) analagous to that seen when vision is interrupted. This may not be possible; although the conditions light versus dark and right eye occluded versus left eye occluded do allow the acquisition of opposite responses, the same sharp generalization decrements may not be found in other modalities (Levinson and Sheridan, 1967a, 1967b). If they are, it would then remain to be demonstrated that drugs achieve response control via actions on these sensory systems.

The possibility that stimulus properties of drugs are mediated by simultaneous effects on several sensory systems is very difficult to test. Individual sensory modalities can be shown not to be *critically* important as above. However, if no individual modality is critical, it is difficult to demonstrate which sensory modalities are involved. It is not feasible to totally deafferent a rat and then train it in a maze. Deletion of a single sensory modality impairs maze learning irrespective of the modality removed. Hence learning curves in partially deafferented rats are often slightly lower than those in intact rats (Woodworth and Schlosberg, 1958, Ch. 21). Such a minor impairment in drug state discriminations after partial deafferentation could be interpreted as indicating that drug discriminations were partially mediated by the interrupted modality. However, as maze learning ability is decreased by deafferentation, the decrement could also occur without any decrease in drug-state distinctiveness. Unless some particular sensory system is primarily responsible for drug-state discriminations, it may not be possible to demonstrate that the sensory systems are involved, even if they are.

SUMMARY

Almost a dozen different types of centrally acting drugs can acquire discriminative control of instrumental responses. Further research may extend the list of active agents. The stimulus properties of these drugs have been compared and contrasted, more extensively in some cases than in others.

Anesthetic drugs have acquired discriminative control in a variety of tasks and species. It is not yet possible to delimit the range of conditions under which these drugs can acquire response control.

The formal rules that describe the characteristics of discriminative control by drugs and by sensory stimuli are strikingly similar. However, peripherally acting drugs and sensory stimuli are generally less effective in acquiring response control than are centrally acting drugs. This argues against the hypothesis that drugs induce distinctive sensory cues that acquire response control through the usual process of sensory discrimination learning. There is no direct evidence to either support or negate the hypothesis that drugs acquire response control by virtue of some central process that is independent of sensory control. Any model proposed to account for response control by drug states must account for the increasing dimensionality of the internal "drug space."

Differences in foot shock intensity do not provide an adequate basis for good discriminative control in the T-maze. However, deletion of visual input does allow rats to readily learn a response antagonistic to the one performed when vision is present. This suggests (but does not demonstrate) that the stimulus properties of drugs could result from a disruption of the normal processes of sensory perception. It also allows us to make a quantitative statement about the magnitude of the stimulus properties of drugs. Apparently for rats, the difference between pentobarbital 15 mg/kg and no drug is about as great as the difference between night and day.

REFERENCES

Ader, R., and Clink, D.W. Effects of chlorpromazine on the acquisition and extinction of an avoidance response in the rat. *J. Pharmacol. Exp. Ther.*, 1957, *121*, 144.

Barnhart, S.S., and Abbott, D.W. Dissociation of learning and meprobamate. *Psychol. Rep.*, 1967, *20*, 520.

Barry, H. Prolonged measurements of discrimination between alcohol and nondrug states. *J. Comp. Physiol. Psychol.*, 1968, *65*, 349.

—— Etheredge, E.E., and Miller, N.E. Counterconditioning and extinction of fear fail to transfer from amobarbital to nondrug state. *Psychopharmacologia (Berl.)*, 1965, *8*, 150.
—— Koepfer, E., and Lutch, J. Learning to discriminate between alcohol and nondrug condition. *Psychol. Rep.*, 1965, *16*, 1072.
—— Miller, N.E., and Tidd, G.E. Control for stimulus change while testing effects of amobarbital on conflict. *J. Comp. Physiol. Psychol.*, 1962, *55*, 1071.
——Wagner, A.R., and Miller, N.E. Effects of alcohol and amobarbital on performance inhibited by experimental extinction. *J. Comp. Physiol. Psychol.*, 1962, *55*, 464.
Belleville, R.E. Control of behavior by drug-produced internal stimuli. *Psychopharmacologia (Berl.)*, 1964, *5*, 95.
Berger, B.D., and Stein, L. An analysis of the learning deficits produced by scopolamine. *Psychopharmacologia (Berl.)*, 1969(a), *14*, 271.
—— and Stein, L. Asymmetrical dissociation of learning between scopolamine and WY4036, a new benzodiazepine tranquilizer. *Psychopharmacologia (Berl.)*, 1969(b), *14*, 351.
Bindra, D., Nyman, K., and Wise, J. Barbiturate-induced dissociation of acquisition and extinction: Role of movement-initiating processes. *J. Comp. Physiol. Psychol.*, 1965, *60*, 223.
—— and Reichert, H. Dissociation of movement initiation without dissociation of response choice. *Psychonomic Science*, 1966, *4*, 95.
—— and Reichert, H. The nature of dissociation: Effects of transitions between normal and barbiturate-induced states on reversal learning and habituation. *Psychopharmacologia (Berl.)*, 1967, *10*, 330.
Bliss, D.K., Sledjeski, M., and Leiman, A. State dependent choice behavior in the rhesus monkey. *Neuropsychologica*, 1970 (In press).
Bohdanecky, Z., and Jarvik, M.E. The effect of d-amphetamine and physostigmine upon acquisition and retrieval in a single trial learning task. *Arch. Int. Pharmacodyn.*, 1967, *170*, 58.
Bradford, J.P., and Macdonald, G.E. Imprinting: Pre- and posttrial administration of pentobarbital and the approach response. *J. Comp. Physiol. Psychol.*, 1969, *68*, 50.
Brown, A., Feldman, R.S., and Moore, J.W. Conditional discrimination learning based on chlordiazepoxide: Dissociation or cue? *J. Comp. Physiol. Psychol.*, 1968, *66*, 211.
Burgoyne, L.M. State dependent learning in the rat. Unpublished M.A. Thesis, McGill University, Montreal, Canada, 1968.
Bustamante, J.A., Jordán, A., Vila, M., Gonzales, A. and Insua, A. State dependent learning in humans. *Physiol. Behav.*, 1970, *5*, 793.
—— Rosselló, A., Jordán, A., Pradera, E., and Insua, A. Learning and drugs. *Physiol. Behav.*, 1968, *3*, 553.
Caird, W.K. An investigation of the effects of alcohol on human learning. Unpublished Progress Report, 1968.
Calhoun, W.H., and Smith, A.A. Effects of scopolamine on acquisition of passive avoidance. *Psychopharmacologia (Berl.)*, 1968, *13*, 201.
Carlson, N.J. The effects of scopolamine on learning, reversal, and rereversal in the T-maze. *Amer. Psychol.*, 1967, *22*, 492. (Abstract)
Carlton, P.L., and Vogel, J.R. Studies of the amnesic properties of scopolamine. *Psychonomic Science*, 1965, *3*, 261.
Caul, W.F. Effects of amobarbital on discrimination acquisition and reversal. *Psychopharmacologia (Berl.)*, 1967, *11*, 414.
Charney, N.H., and Reynolds, G.S. Tolerance to the behavioral effects of scopolamine in rats. *Psychopharmacologia (Berl.)*, 1967, *11*, 379.
Chen, Chia-Shong. A study of the alcohol-tolerance effect and an introduction of a new behavioral technique. *Psychopharmacologia (Berl.)*, 1968, *12*, 433.

Cicala, G.A., and Hartley, D.L. Drugs and the learning and performance of fear. *J. Comp. Physiol. Psychol.*, 1967, *64*, 175.

Conger, J.J. The effect of alcohol on conflict behavior in the albino rat. *Quart. J. Stud. Alcohol*, 1951, *12*, 1.

Cook, L., Davidson, A., Davis, D.J., and Kelleher, R.T. Epinephrine, norepinephrine, and acetylcholine as conditioned stimuli for avoidance behavior. *Science*, 1960, *131*, 990.

Crow, L.T. Effects of alcohol on conditioned avoidance responding. *Physiol. Behav.*, 1966, *1*, 89.

—— Alcohol state transfer effects with performance maintained by intracranial self-stimulation. *Physiol. Behav.*, 1970, *5*, 515.

Daly, H.B. Disruptive effects of scopolamine on fear conditioning and on instrumental escape learning. *J. Comp. Physiol. Psychol.*, 1968, *66*, 579.

Doty, L.A., and Doty, B.A. Chlorpromazine-produced response decrements as a function of problem difficulty level. *J. Comp. Physiol. Psychol.*, 1963, *56*, 740.

Evans, H.L., and Patton, R.A. Scopolamine effects on a one-trial test of fear conditioning. *Psychonomic Science*, 1968, *11*, 229.

Gardner, L. and McCollough, C. A reinvestigation of the dissociative effects of curareform drugs. *Amer. Psychol.*, 1962, *17*, 398. (Abstract)

Giarman, N.J., and Pepeu, G. The influence of centrally acting cholinolytic drugs on brain acetylcholine levels. *Brit. J. Pharmacol.*, 1964, *23*, 123.

Girden, E. Cerebral mechanisms in conditioning under curare. *Amer. J. Psychol.*, 1940, *53*, 397.

—— and Culler, E.A. Conditioned responses in curarized striate muscle in dogs. *J. Comp. Psychol.*, 1937, *23*, 261.

Goodwin, D.W., Powell, B., Bremer, D., Haine, H., and Stern, J. Alcohol and recall: State dependent effects in man. *Science*, 1969, *163*, 1358.

Grossman, S.P., and Miller, N.E. Control for stimulus-change in the evaluation of alcohol and chlorpromazine as fear-reducing drugs. *Psychopharmacologia (Berl.)*, 1961, *2*, 342.

Gruber, R.P., Stone, G.C., and Reed, D.R. Scopolamine-induced anterograde amnesia. *Int. J. Neuropharmacol.*, 1967, *6*, 187.

Harris, R.T., and Balster, R.L. Discriminative control of dl-amphetamine and saline of lever choice and response patterning. *Psychonomic Science*, 1968, *10*, 105.

—— and Balster, R.L. An analysis of the function of drugs in the stimulus control of operant behavior. In Thompson, T., and Pickens, R., eds., *Stimulus Properties of Drugs*. New York, Appleton-Century-Crofts, 1971.

Heistad, G.T. A bio-psychological approach to somatic treatments in psychiatry. *Amer. J. Psychiat.*, 1957, *114*, 540.

—— Effects of chlorpromazine and electro-convulsive shock on a conditioned emotional response. *J. Comp. Physiol. Psychol.*, 1958, *51*, 209.

—— and Torres, A.A. A mechanism for the effect of a tranquilizing drug on learned emotional responses. *University of Minnesota Medical Bulletin*, 1959, *30*, 518.

Hill, H.E., Jones, E., and Bell, E.C. State dependent control of discrimination by morphine and pentobarbital. NIMH Addiction Research Center, Lexington, Ky., 1970 (In preparation).

Holmgren, B. Conditional avoidance reflex under pentobarbital. *Bol. Inst. Estud. Med. Biol. (Mexico)*, 1964, *22*, 21.

—— Drug dependent conditioned reflexes. Paper read at International Symposium on Cortical-Subcortical Relationships in Sensory Regulation. Havana, Cuba, 1965.

Iwahara, S., Iwasaki, T., and Hasegawa, Y. Effects of chlorpromazine and homofenazine upon a passive avoidance response in rats. *Psychopharmacologia (Berl.)*, 1968, *13*, 320.

—— Nagamura, N., and Iwasaki, T. Effect of chlordiazepoxide upon experimental extinction in the straight runway as a function of partial reinforcement in the rat. *Japanese Psychological Research*, 1967, *9*, 128.

Kamano, D.K., and Arp, D.J. Effects of chlordiazepoxide (Librium) on the acquisition and extinction of avoidance responses. *Psychopharmacologia (Berl.)*, 1964, *6*, 112.

Kanzler, A.W. Effect of alcohol on the conditioned emotional response of the albino rat. Unpublished M.A. Thesis, California State College, Long Beach, 1967.

Kubena, R.K., and Barry, H. Two procedures for training differential responses in alcohol and nondrug conditions. *J. Pharm. Sci.*, 1969, *58*, 99.

Kurland, H.D., Cassell, S., and Goldberg, E.M. The effects of chlorpromazine on the transferability of learning in humans. Paper read at Society of Biological Psychiatry, Washington, D.C., 1968.

Lal, H. Control of learned conditioned-avoidance responses (CAR) by amphetamine and chlorpromazine. *Psychopharmacologia (Berl.)* 1969, *14*, 33.

Leiman, A.L., Bliss, D.K., Powers, J.B., and Rosenzweig, M.R. Electrical correlates of drug-dissociated learning. *Fed. Proc.*, 1967, *26*, 263. (Abstract)

Levinson, D.M., and Sheridan, C.L. Retention in guinea pigs of monocular pattern discriminations during reversal acquisition with the opposite eye. *Psychonomic Science*, 1967(a), *7*, 239.

―― and Sheridan, C.L. Acquisition and retention of monocular discriminations in rats as a function of relevant (reversal) or irrelevant opposite-eye training. *Psychonomic Science*, 1967(b), *8*, 475.

Longo, V.G. Behavioral and electroencephalographic effects of atropine and related compounds. *Pharmacol. Rev.*, 1966, *18*, 965.

Madill, M.F. Alcohol-induced dissociation in humans: A possible treatment technique for alcoholism. Unpublished Ph.D. Thesis, University of Toronto, 1967.

Marriott, A.S., and Spencer, P.S.J. Effects of centrally acting drugs on exploratory behavior in rats. *Brit. J. Pharmacol.*, 1965, *25*, 432.

Meyers, B. Some effects of scopolamine on a passive-avoidance response in rats. *Psychopharmacologia (Berl.)*, 1965, *8*, 111.

Moffett, A., and Ettlinger, G. Opposite responding to position in the light and dark. *Neuropsychologia*, 1967, *5*, 59.

Oliverio, A. Effects of scopolamine on avoidance conditioning of mice. *Psychopharmacologia (Berl.)*, 1968, *12*, 214.

Osborn, A.G., Bunker, J.P., Cooper, L.M., Frank, G.S., and Hilgard, E.R. Effects of thiopental sedation on learning and memory. *Science*, 1967, *157*, 574.

Otis, L.S. Dissociation and recovery of a response learned under the influence of chlorpromazine or saline. *Science*, 1964, *143*, 1347.

Overton, D.A. State-dependent or "dissociated" learning produced with pentobarbital. *J. Comp. Physiol. Psychol.*, 1964, *57*, 3.

―― State-dependent learning produced by depressant and atropine-like drugs. *Psychopharmacologia (Berl.)*, 1966, *10*, 6.

―― Differential responding in a three choice maze controlled by three drug states. *Psychopharmacologia (Berl.)*, 1967, *11*, 376.

―― Visual cues and shock sensitivity in the control of T maze choice by drug conditions. *J. Comp. Physiol. Psychol.*, 1968(a), *66*, 216.

―― Dissociated learning in drug states (state-dependent learning). In Efron, D.H. *et al.*, eds., *Psychopharmacology. A review of progress*. PHS Publication #1836, U.S. Government Printing Office, Washington, D.C., 918, 1968(b).

―― Control of T-maze choice by nicotinic, antinicotinic and antimuscarinic drugs. Proceedings 77th Annual Convention of American Psychological Association, 1969, 869.

Paskal, V. Dissociative effects of atropine on a simple learned task in the rat. *Undergraduate Research Reports in Psychology*, McGill University, Montreal, Canada, 37, 1962. (Briefly described in Overton, 1968b).

Phillips, S.M. An analysis of state-dependent learning. Unpublished M.A. Thesis, University of California, Davis, California, 1967.

Ross, D.G. Relationship of method of drug withdrawal to resulting amount of response disruption in reversal learning. Unpublished M.A. Thesis, Bradley University, Peoria, Illinois, 1967.

Rushton, R., Steinberg, H., and Tinson, C. Effects of a single experience on subsequent reactions to drugs. *Brit. J. Pharmacol.*, 1963, 20, 99.

Ryback, R. State dependent or "dissociated" learning with alcohol in the goldfish. *Quart. J. Stud. Alcohol*, 1969, 30, 598.

Sachs, E., Weingarten, M., and Klein, N.W., Jr. Effects of chlordiazepoxide on the acquisition of avoidance learning and its transfer to the normal state and other drug conditions. *Psychopharmacologia (Berl.)*, 1966, 9, 17.

Schuster, C.R., and Brady, J.V. The discriminate control of a food-reinforced operant by interoceptive stimulation. In Thompson, T. and Pickens, R., eds., *Stimulus Properties of Drugs*. New York, Appleton-Century-Crofts, 1971.

Seymore, J.D. The effect of ethyl alcohol in producing state dependent or "dissociated" learning in rats. M.S. Thesis, Department of Psychology, University of Southern Mississippi, 1967.

Sherman, A.R. Therapy of maladaptive fear-motivated behavior in the rat by systematic withdrawal of a fear-reducing drug. *Behav. Res. Ther.*, 1967, 5, 121.

Shillito, E.E. The effect of chlorpromazine and thioridazine on the exploration of a Y maze by rats. *Brit. J. Pharmacol.*, 1967, 30, 258.

Shmavonian, B.H. Effects of Serpasil (Rauwolfia serpentina) on fear training. Unpublished M.A. Thesis, University of Washington, Seattle, Washington, 1956.

Solomon, R.L., and Turner, L.H. Discriminative classical conditioning in dogs paralyzed by curare can later control discriminative avoidance responses in the normal state. *Psychol. Rev.*, 1962, 66, 202.

Stark, L. The inability of scopolamine to induce state-dependent one-trial learning. *Fed. Proc.*, 1967, 26, 613. (Abstract)

Stewart, J. Differential responses based on the physiological consequences of pharmacological agents. *Psychopharmacologia (Berl.)*, 1963, 3, 132.

Storm, T., and Caird, W.K. The effects of alcohol on serial verbal learning in chronic alcoholics. *Psychonomic Science*, 1967, 9, 43.

Tarter, R.E. Dissociative effects of ethyl alcohol. M.A. Thesis, Department of Psychology, Dalhousie University. Halifax, Nova Scotia, Canada, 1968.

Tenen, S.S. Recovery time as a measure of CER strength: Effects of benzodiazepines, amobarbital, chlorpromazine and amphetamine. *Psychopharmacologia (Berl.)*, 1967, 12, 1.

Vogel, J.R., Hughes, R.A., and Carlton, P.L. Scopolamine, atropine, and conditioned fear. *Psychopharmacologia (Berl.)*, 1967, 10, 409.

White, R.P., Nash, C.B., Westerbeke, E.J., and Possanza, G.J. Phylogenetic comparison of central actions produced by different doses of atropine and hyoscine. *Arch. Int. Pharmacodyn.*, 1961, 132, 349.

Woodworth, R.S., and Schlosberg, H. *Experimental Psychology*. New York, Holt and Co., 1958.

7

An Analysis of the Function of Drugs in the Stimulus Control of Operant Behavior[1]

Robert T. Harris and Robert L. Balster[2]

Behavioral Pharmacology Section
Texas Research Institute,
Houston, Texas

Only in recent years have CNS-active drugs been found to act effectively as discriminative stimuli in the control of learned behavior. A recent review (Overton, 1968) noted that many classes of drugs have been successfully employed to exert discriminative control over behavior, across a variety of tasks, e.g., T-mazes (Overton, 1964, 1966; Barry, Koepfer, and Lutch, 1965), shuttle boxes (Bindra, Nyman, and Wise, 1965), conditioned fear situations (Heistad and Torres, 1959), and operant techniques (Barry and Kubena, 1967; Harris and Balster, 1968), and for a variety of reinforcers, e.g., food (Barry et al., 1965), water (Korman, Knopf, and Leon, 1963), and shock (Overton, 1966). Thus, the generality of the discriminative stimulus function of drugs has been adequately established.

A relative assessment of the sensitivity of various behavioral parameters to stimulus control by drugs, however, is difficult to obtain from experimental situations as diverse as these. Of considerable methodological importance to the analysis of drug-stimulus control would be studies in which the major parameters of operantly conditioned behavior are examined systematically. In the present experiments, such an analysis was attempted, with the same basic operant technique employed to investigate the factors which control drug-discriminated behavior. The behavioral parameters studied included reinforcement schedules with different reinforcing stimuli, drug-

---

[1] This research was partially supported by USPHS Research Grant No. MH 14434. The authors wish to thank June Taylor, Dale Box, and especially Patti Stump for their assistance in conducting these experiments.
[2] Partially supported by USAF Contract F2900-c-0014 with 6571st Aeromedical Research Laboratory, Holloman AFB, Alamogordo, New Mexico.

generalization relationships with transfer and dose-response effects, drug-discrimination reversals, and drug-probe functions. A single drug, *dl*-amphetamine, was also used throughout the study, although several additional drugs were included in many of the experiments.

EXPERIMENTAL PROCEDURE

All investigations were carried out with female Sprague-Dawley rats. The apparatus was operant conditioning chambers equipped with either one or two response levers located on a front stimulus panel. The basic procedure involved training the animals on a two-component multiple (mult) reinforcement schedule, in which each schedule component was indicated by a specific (drug or saline) discriminative stimulus. The schedule components alternated randomly from day to day. Both one- and two-lever procedures were used. For one-lever procedures, both schedule components were programmed on the same cage lever; for two-lever procedures, responding on one cage lever produced reinforcement on one schedule component and responding on a second cage lever produced reinforcement on the other schedule component. On two-lever procedures, to prevent chaining of responses between the two levers, a response on the incorrect lever during the one schedule component either reset the timing interval on temporal schedules or did not step the response counter on ratio schedules. Each daily session was one hour in duration. The reinforcer was either a 45-mg Noyes food pellet or shock delivered through the grid floor of the chamber. Between sessions the animals were returned to their home cages and fed for one hour immediately after the experimental session. Drug injections were given 15 minutes prior to each session.

Following training under each of two drug states, tests for stimulus control were made during extinction with the drugs used during training, or with other drugs or drug doses. At least six reinforcement sessions preceded each test condition.

The results for each procedure are presented as cumulative records for one animal, selected as representative of the animals trained and tested under that condition. On the records, lever responses are recorded cumulatively, with reinforcements indicated by diagonal slashes of the recording pen. For two-lever procedures, incorrect lever responses are indicated by marks on the event pen. Each record indicates, numerically, the total number of responses on each schedule component for the entire one-hour session, although the records, as shown, present only the first 15 or 25 minutes of the session.

FOOD REINFORCEMENT SCHEDULES

A multiple reinforcement schedule involving differential reinforcement of low response rate (DRL) and/or fixed-ratio (FR) reinforcement components was used. On FR schedules, reinforcement follows a fixed number of responses, and on DRL schedules, reinforcement occurs when responses are separated by a fixed period of time.

DRL schedules possess several advantages for drug discrimination procedures: reinforcement density is low, thus minimizing anorexic effects of drugs; response frequency is low, thus minimizing activity impedance; responding in extinction is prolonged; and, responding occurs at approximately equal rates, thus providing quantitative comparisons of the extent of control exercised by any two drug combinations.

FR schedules are useful when response rate is important in analyzing the stimulus control of drugs during extinction. The characteristic bursts of responses followed by periods of post-reinforcement pausing engendered by this schedule can be easily distinguished from patterns of responding reflective of other histories of reinforcement. With ratio schedules, occasional difficulty is encountered in training an animal to a sustained high rate under chronic drug treatment, particularly the psychomotor stimulants.

Controls. Of considerable importance in analyzing the stimulus control of drugs when the components of a schedule are changed from day to day is the way in which responding develops in the absence of programmed stimulus control or under the control of external stimuli. Thus, control procedures were used which involved training the animals on a two-component mixed (mix) reinforcement schedule, in which no discriminative stimuli were associated with each schedule component, or on a two-component multiple reinforcement schedule with external stimuli serving as discriminative stimuli for each component.

Figure 1 shows the cumulative records of the 35th day of reinforcement for each component of a mix FR 50 DRL 20-sec schedule, and subsequent extinction tests. During FR reinforcement, responding occurred almost entirely on the reinforced lever, thus demonstrating that the reinforcing stimulus functioned as an effective discriminative stimulus. This was not the case during DRL reinforcement, however, where frequent bursts of responses occurred on the incorrect (FR) lever. During the two extinction sessions presented in Figure 1, the animal responded on each lever at the rate appropriate to previous reinforcement on that lever. Frequent alternation

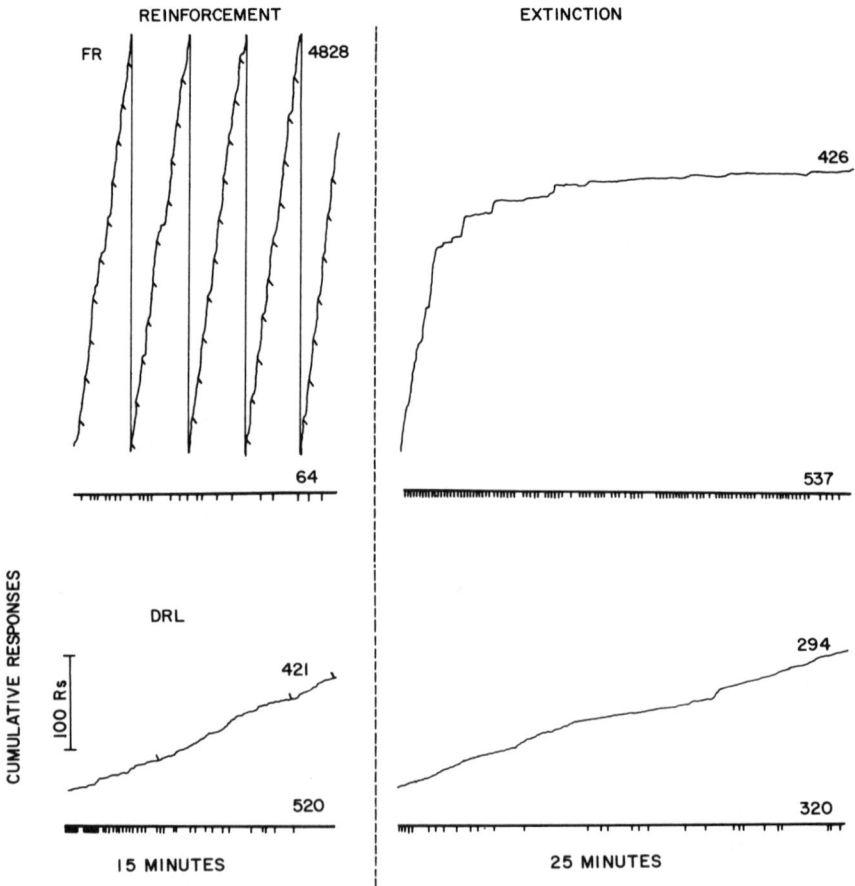

Fig. 1. Two-lever mix FR 50 DRL 20-sec food reinforcement and extinction.

between the levers occurred which indicated that any position or schedule preference that might have existed did not markedly influence the distribution of responses during extinction.

Figure 2 presents reinforcement and extinction records for responses of a two-lever mix FR 50 FR 50 schedule. In this case, responding on the correct lever during reinforcement was not as well controlled by the reinforcing stimulus as was previously shown for the mix FR DRL schedule (Fig. 1). Responding during extinction was approximately evenly distributed between the two levers, again indicating that response probing on both levers is the predominate behavior of an animal performing in the absence of discriminative stimuli.

Figure 3 presents cumulative records for an animal trained on a two-lever

An Analysis of the Function of Drugs 115

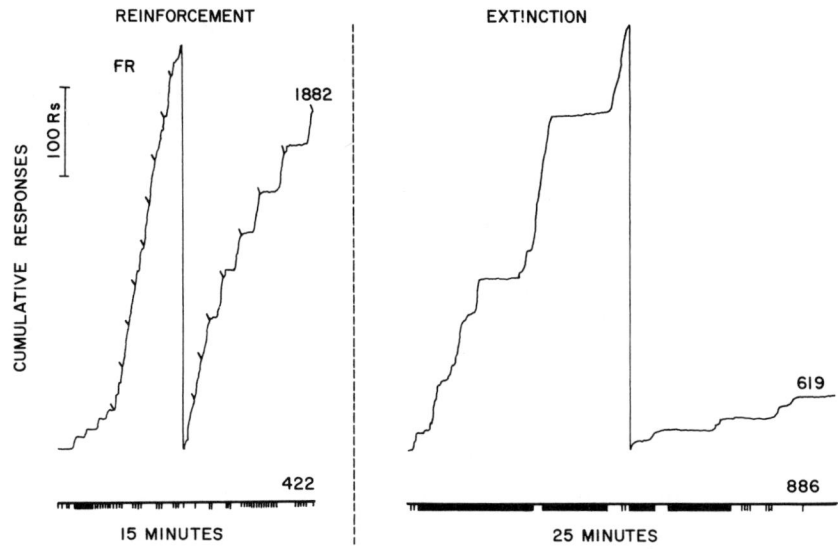

Fig. 2. Two-lever mix FR 50 FR 50 food reinforcement and extinction.

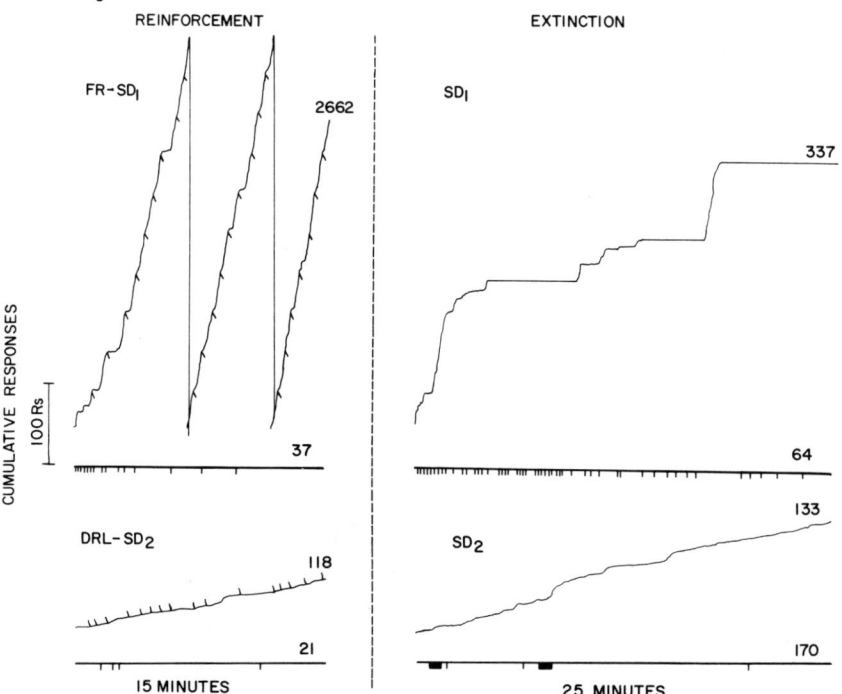

Fig. 3. Two-lever mult FR 50 DRL 20-sec food reinforcement and extinction.

mult FR 50 DRL 20-sec schedule with external stimuli (SD) programmed with each schedule component. SD_1 was bright illumination provided by two lights mounted over the levers and indicated FR reinforcement, and SD_2 was dim illumination provided by a small house light and indicated DRL reinforcement.

Responding during reinforcement was satisfactorily controlled by the reinforcers and/or changes in illumination. Responding in extinction was less clearly under stimulus control. During FR extinction under SD_1, responding on the DRL lever (recorded on event pen) occurred throughout the session, and although the ratio of correct to incorrect responses (337/64) was in the direction of the stimulus-associated lever, stimulus control by bright light cannot be considered strong because the response total on that lever could be expected to supersede the total count on the DRL lever. Similarly, the performance during DRL extinction under SD_2 does not reflect strong discriminative control by dim light. While lever presses on the DRL lever predominated throughout the session, sufficient bursts of responding occurred on the FR lever to produce a greater response total (133/170). These results indicate that external stimuli exercise some degree of discriminative control over responding in multiple schedules where the components of the schedule are changed from day to day.

The records for the mixed and externally controlled multiple schedules provide a basis for comparison of the effectiveness of drugs as discriminative stimuli.

Drugs as discriminative stimuli. Initially, drugs were used as discriminative stimuli on a two-lever, multiple continuous reinforcement (CRF) schedule (mult CRF CRF). *dl*-Amphetamine sulfate (1.0 mg/kg) and saline were the discriminative stimuli for each schedule component. No drug discrimination effect could be obtained on this schedule. Responding during reinforcement was under the strong stimulus control of the reinforcer, as in the case of FR reinforcement (Fig. 3). During extinction, responding was distributed approximately evenly between the two levers.[3]

Figure 4 shows the performance of a rat reinforced on a two-lever DRL 20-sec DRL 20-sec schedule of reinforcement. Ethyl alcohol (1,200 mg/kg) and saline (12.0 ml/kg) were used as discriminative stimuli for responding on each schedule. Extinction records following the 13th day of training under ethanol and 20th day under saline are presented. In both cases, responding

---

[3]External stimuli, in this case the presence or absence of a clicking sound, also proved ineffective as discriminative stimuli during extinction. A possible explanation for these results may be that during reinforcement on CRF the reinforcer itself is a sufficiently powerful stimulus to mask the effects of other stimuli programmed into the environment.

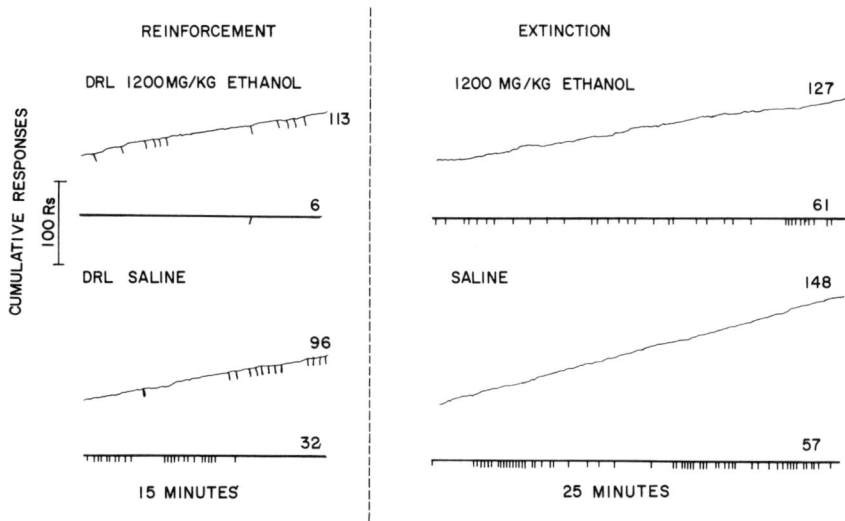

Fig. 4. Two-lever mult DRL 20-sec DRL 20-sec food reinforcement and extinction.

during extinction occurred primarily on the lever associated with the appropriate drug state during reinforcement.

Ethanol did not function as well as other drugs used on this schedule in that incorrect responses (error) during both reinforcement and extinction were high; whereas, with other drugs (*dl*-amphetamine, atropine) as few as 10 to 15 errors were common for most extinction records.

Figure 5 shows the performance of a rat trained on a two-lever mult FR 50 FR 50 schedule. Atropine sulfate (9.0 mg/kg) and methyl atropine nitrate (12.0 mg/kg) were used as discriminative stimuli. The extinction records follow the 17th day of training under atropine and the 21st day under methyl atropine. Responding during reinforcement was not impeded by either drug, with either few or no incorrect lever responses. Responding during extinction under both drugs occurred at the high rate characteristic of a ratio schedule with increasingly longer periods of no responding appearing later in the session.

The difference in control exerted by methyl atropine and atropine reflects the tendency for all subjects, under any drug condition, to vary somewhat in their response patterns during repeated extinction periods. The same factor can be considered to apply to the differences in errors shown under each drug.

Figure 6 shows the performance of three subjects trained on a two-lever

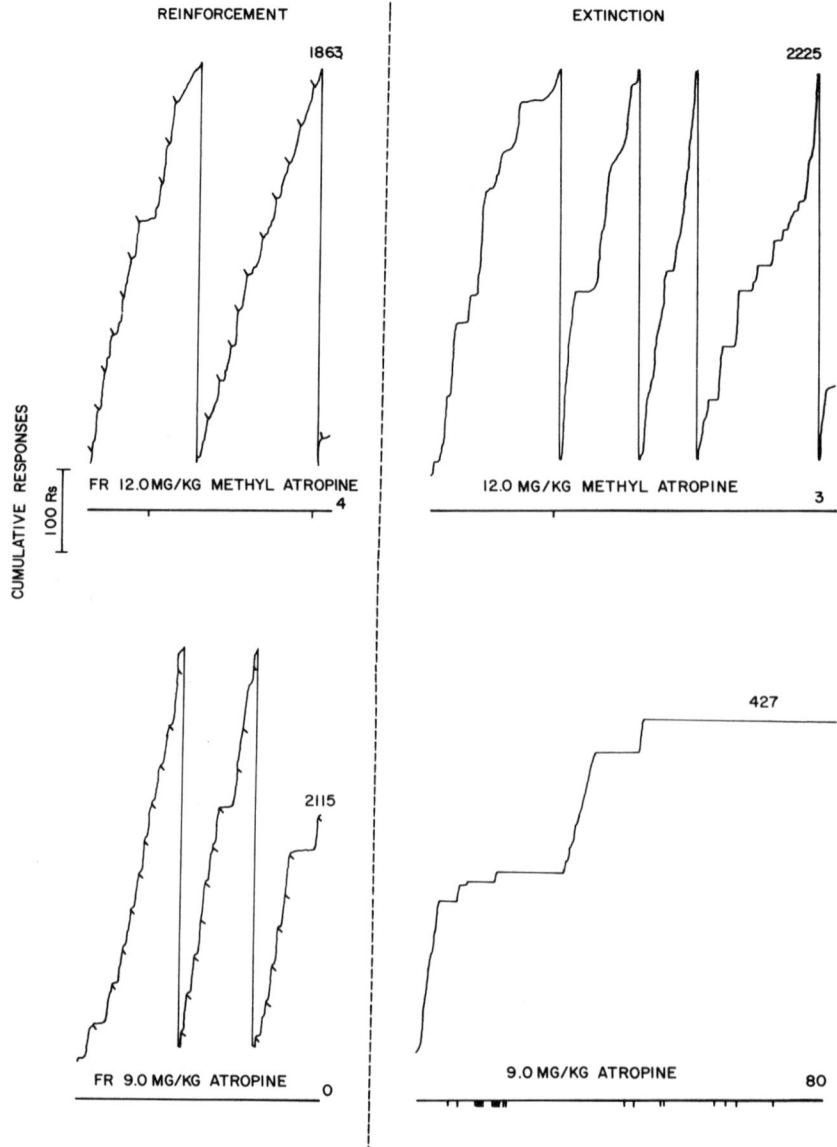

Fig. 5. Two-lever mult FR 50 FR 50 food reinforcement and extinction.

mult FR 50 DRL 20-sec schedule, with saline (1.0 ml/kg) as the discriminative stimulus for FR reinforcement and *dl*-amphetamine sulfate (1.0 mg/kg)

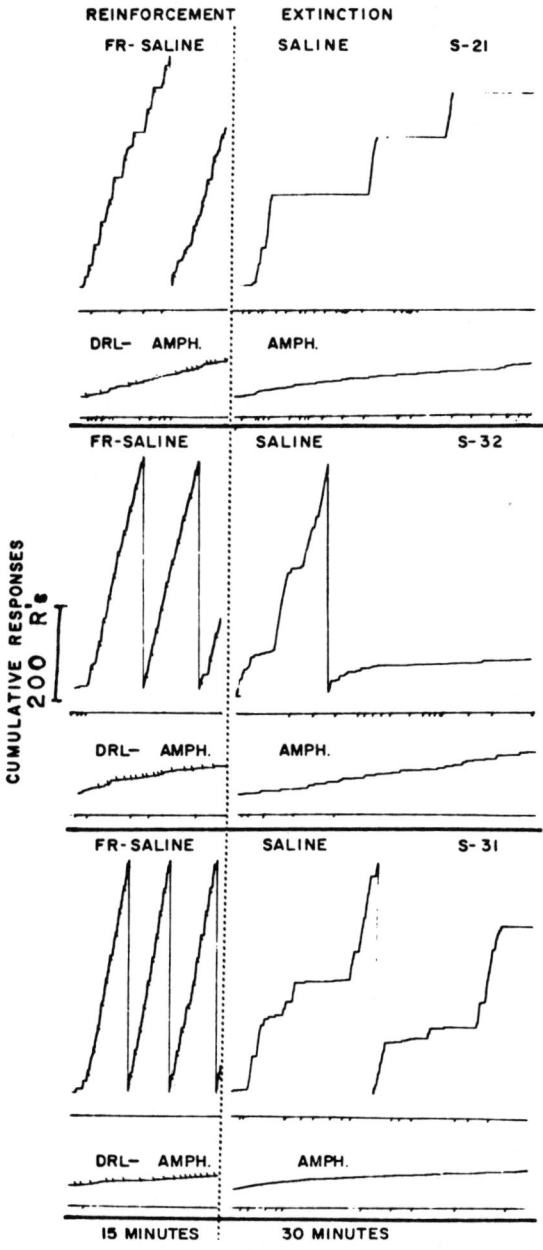

Fig. 6. Two-lever mult FR 50 DRL 20-sec food reinforcement and extinction.

as the discriminative stimulus for DRL reinforcement. Extinction occurred following eight days of training under each drug state.

As can be seen, responding in extinction corresponded to the drug condition of training. Response patterning also appeared to be under the stimulus control of each drug state. In view of the fact that each lever can be considered to have exercised some degree of control over the rate at which it is pressed (see Fig. 1), the question of whether drugs alone can control response patterning in addition to lever choice awaits a condition in which a single lever is used.

A major advantage of the mult FR DRL schedule, and perhaps any multiple schedule comprised of two widely different contingencies, is the rapidity with which discriminative control can be established. Multiple schedules comprised of different schedule components are limited when quantitative (response frequency) comparisons of stimulus control are desired. Marked differences in rates or pause durations between divergent schedule components preclude tabular representation of the data. Cumulative records appear to be the most meaningful manner in which stimulus control during extinction can be shown. For example, on several occasions the subjects emitted bursts of responses on the FR lever when extinguished under the DRL drug state (amphetamine). On the one hand, the response totals for these sessions showed more incorrect than correct responses, which would suggest an absence of stimulus control by the drug. On the other hand, the length of time that the subject responded on the correct lever would indicate that the drug exercised considerable stimulus control over the animal's behavior.

Figure 7 presents cumulative records of an animal trained on a mult FR 50 DRL 20-sec schedule in which only one lever was used, and schedule components alternated on a daily basis. Saline (1.0 ml/kg) and dl-amphetamine (1.0 mg/kg) were used as discriminative stimuli for each schedule component. The response rate during DRL reinforcement was higher than the rate ordinarily obtained from animals trained only on DRL schedules, which probably reflects an inductive effect from the FR component of the schedule. This effect is not observed in two-lever mult FR DRL schedules. Responding during extinction corresponded closely to the rate obtained during reinforcement under each drug state, which demonstrates that drug states can exercise discriminative control over response patterns as well as over lever choice. In comparison to two-lever tests using the same schedule components (Fig. 6), the control of drug states over response patterning may be considered superior to that over lever choice. Responding throughout the amphetamine extinction session was characteristic of DRL reinforcement, and only a few segments of spaced responding appear in the saline extinction

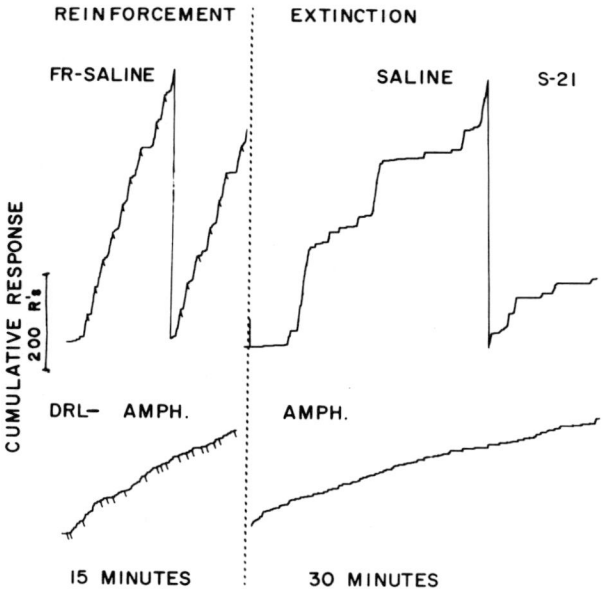

Fig. 7. One-lever mult FR 50 DRL 20-sec food reinforcement and extinction.

record. In two-lever tests, on the other hand, responding occurs sporadically on the incorrect lever.

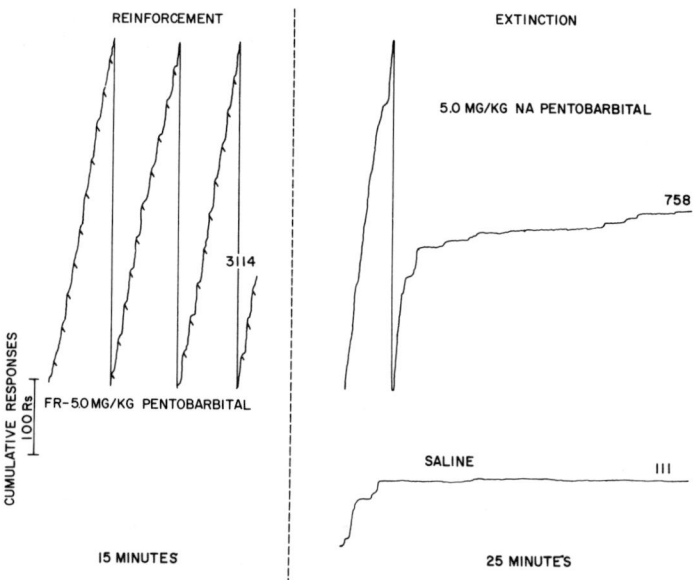

Fig. 8. One-lever mult FR 50 EXT food reinforcement and extinction.

Figure 8 presents cumulative records of a rat trained on a one-lever mult FR 50 extinction (EXT) schedule. Saline (1.0 ml/kg) for the EXT component and sodium pentobarbital (5.0 mg/kg) for the FR component were used as discriminative stimuli. The extinction record under pentobarbital reflects the previous history of FR reinforcement under the same drug state. The saline record shows FR bursts of responding during the first five minutes of the session, followed by complete extinction.

Two other animals were trained on this schedule, using *dl*-amphetamine (1.0 mg/kg) for the EXT component and saline for the FR component as discriminative stimuli (data not graphically presented). In this case, extinction under saline following FR reinforcement was similar to that shown in Figure 8 for pentobarbital; however, extinction under amphetamine was considerably faster than shown for saline.

SHOCK-AVOIDANCE REINFORCEMENT SCHEDULES

Figure 9 shows performance during reinforcement and extinction of animals trained on a nondiscriminative (Sidman) avoidance schedule on either of two levers, both of which were programmed on the same temporal contingency (RS = 35 sec, SS = 5 sec). *dl*-Amphetamine (1.0 mg/kg) and

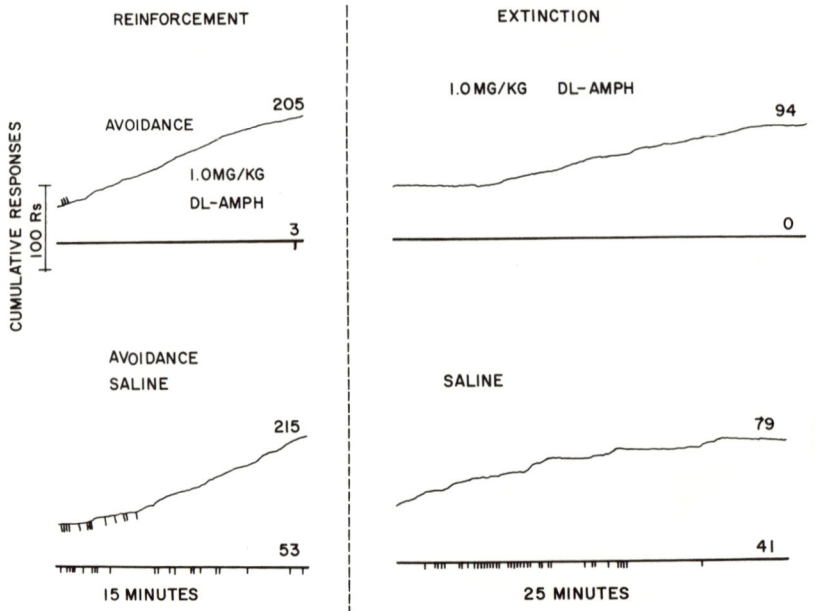

Fig. 9. Two-lever mult avoidance-avoidance shock reinforcement and extinction.

saline (1.0 ml/kg) were used as discriminative stimuli for responding on each lever for shock avoidance. Under amphetamine, responding during both reinforcement and extinction was almost entirely on the appropriate lever and at a rate which avoided shock deliveries. The early shocks shown on the reinforcement record can be considered a "warm-up" effect. Under saline, on the other hand, responding during reinforcement and extinction was considerably more distributed between the two levers. This phenomenon was observed in the records of two other animals trained under identical conditions. Strong stimulus control by drugs was obtained more rapidly and attained a higher degree of accuracy with shock-avoidance schedules than was the case with positively reinforced schedules. One reason for this may be that the relative absence of shock during effective avoidance minimizes its importance as a discriminative stimulus during training. Further, extinction is very similar to reinforcement on avoidance schedules where the animal is responding steadily, thus incorrect responding does not occur as it does on food-reinforced schedules.

IMPLICATIONS OF RESULTS

Table 1 summarizes the results of schedule comparisons. These results demonstrate that the stimulus function of drugs is not peculiar to specific schedule or reinforcement parameters. Further, they reveal a near equivalence of drug effectiveness in controlling schedules of reinforcement, and indicate that schedule-induced rate of responding may be more sensitive to drug stimulus control than choice behavior.

The relationship between the pharmacologic activity of a drug and its effects on behavior can be viewed differently from that found in standard "screening" tests when a drug is employed as a discriminative stimulus. For example, in the present study tolerance did not develop (in a behavioral sense) even though the drugs were administered three times per week over a period of three to five months. To be sure, pharmacologic tolerance may not have occurred either. In any event, the fact that the stimulus control function of a wide class of drugs did not vary with chronic administration suggests that drug tolerance of pharmacologic systems may not be manifested in the mechanisms responsible for stimulus control.

Again, it was possible with several drugs to produce an effect on behavior that was descriptively opposite to that noted in pharmacologic assays, e.g., pentobarbital-induced FR response bursts and amphetamine-induced DRL pacing during extinction. These paradoxes are not presented as refutations of pharmacologic taxonomies of drug action but, rather, as cautions that need

Table 1. *Training schedule and results*

Schedule	Drugs	Result	Number of Subjects
Two-lever mult CRF CRF	1.0 MG/KG dl-Amphetamine Sulfate 1.0 ML/KG Saline	N.C.[a]	2
Two-lever mult DRL DRL	1.0 MG/KG dl-Amphetamine Sulfate 1.0 ML/KG Saline	Strong[b]	1
Two-lever mult DRL DRL	1200 MG/KG Ethanol 12 ML/KG Saline	Strong	1
Two-lever mult DRL DRL	1.0 MG/KG Chlorpromazine Hydrochloride 1.0 Saline	N.C.	1
Two-lever mult FR FR	1.0 MG/KG dl-Amphetamine Sulfate 1.0 ML/KG Saline	Strong	2
Two-lever mult FR FR	1.0 MG/KG dl-Amphetamine Sulfate 1.0 MG/KG Chlorpromazine Hydrochloride	Strong	1
Two-lever mult FR FR	10.0 MG/KG Atropine Sulfate 1.0 ML/KG Saline	Strong Weak[c]	3 1
Two-lever mult FR FR	10.0 MG/KG Methyl Atropine Nitrate 1.0 ML/KG Saline	N.C.	1
Two-lever mult FR FR	10.00 MG/KG Atropine Sulfate 12.00 MG/KG Methyl Atropine Nitrate	Strong	2
Two-lever mult FR FR	1.0 MG/KG dl-Amphetamine 4.5 MG/KG Methylphenidate Hydrochloride	N.C.	1
Two-lever mult FR FR	0.4 MG/KG Psilocybin 1.0 ML/KG Saline	Weak	2
Two-lever mult FR FR	0.2 MG/KG Psilocybin 0.025 MG/KG LSD-25	N.C.	2
Two-lever mult FR FR	25.0 MG/KG Chlordiazepoxide Hydrochloride 1.0 ML/KG Saline	Strong	1
Two-lever mult FR FR	1.0 MG/KG Chlorpromazine Hydrochloride 1.0 MG/KG Chlorprothixene	N.C.	1
Two-lever mult FR DRL	1.0 MG/KG dl-Amphetamine Sulfate 1.0 ML/KG Saline	Strong	9
Two-lever mult Avoid-Avoid	1.0 MG/KG dl-Amphetamine Sulfate 1.0 ML/KG Saline	Strong	2
One-lever mult FR EXT	1.0 MG/KG dl-Amphetamine Sulfate 1.0 ML/KG Saline	Strong	2
One-lever mult FR EXT	1.0 MG/KG dl-Amphetamine Sulfate 1.0 MG/KG Chlorpromazine Hydrochloride	Strong	1
One-lever mult FR EXT	5.0 MG/KG Sodium Pentobarbital 1.0 ML/KG Saline	Strong	1
One-lever mult FR DRL	1.0 MG/KG dl-Amphetamine Sulfate 1.0 ML/KG Saline	Strong	5
One-lever mult FR DRL	2.0 MG/KG Chlorpromazine Hydrochloride 2.0 ML/KG Saline	N.C.	1

[a] extinction comparable to mixed schedule
[b] extinction showing better control than external stimuli
[c] extinction showing control comparable to external stimuli

to be observed when interpretations of the behavioral effects of drugs are predicated on their pharmacologic activity.

In view of the fact that most drugs employed in therapeutic environments or self-administered in social complexes possess marked CNS activity, the phenomenon of stimulus control may not be restricted to the experimental setting.

In the present experimental paradigm, the finding of greater potency of drugs than illumination differences to act as discriminative stimuli does not warrant generalizations to other external stimuli or other experimental tasks. Nevertheless, we believe that further investigations will confirm the differences shown. Drugs can be thought to be more effective than external events as discriminative stimuli for at least two reasons. First, they are unique to the organism. Generalizations to stimulus sources emanating from the experimental setting or living quarters are less likely to occur with drugs than with sounds or lights. Second, drugs are pervasive and intense in their action. Animals cannot attenuate the stimulus properties of drugs in the manner possible with external stimuli, for example, by changing position or closing their eyes.

GENERALIZATION

Figure 10 presents cumulative records of DRL responding by an animal trained on a one-lever mult FR 50 DRL 20-sec schedule in which dl-amphetamine (1.0 mg/kg) was the discriminative stimulus for DRL reinforcement and saline (1.0 ml/kg) was the discriminative stimulus for FR reinforcement. DRL reinforcement produced the typically low, spaced response pattern which is characteristic of that schedule. DRL extinction at 1.0 mg/kg (upper right panel) produced a record similar to that of reinforcement. A test generalization dose of 0.5 mg/kg (lower left panel) produced an extinction record that combined segments of DRL rates with short bursts of responses representative of FR extinction. A test dose of 0.3 mg/kg (lower right panel) produced an FR extinction record comparable to that obtained after saline injections. Generally, ordered dose-response relationships could only be obtained with the training dose, a minimally effective dose, and a dose midway between the two. This was probably due to the relatively low doses used in these studies.

Figure 11 shows the results of extinction tests with drugs other than the one used as a discriminative stimulus during reinforcement training. The animal had been trained on a one-lever mult FR 50 EXT schedule with dl-amphetamine (1.0 mg/kg) as the discriminative stimulus for FR reinforcement and saline (1.0 ml/kg) for extinction. Extinction sessions with methylphenidate hydrochloride (4.5 mg/kg) or d-amphetamine (1.0 mg/kg) resulted in responding at the high rate characteristic of extinction after FR training,

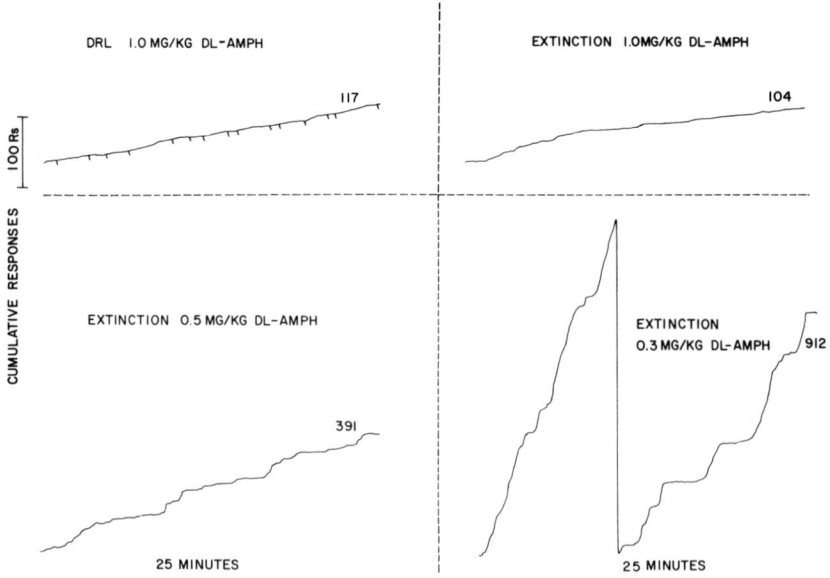

Fig. 10. Dose-response generalization. One-lever mult FR 50 DRL 20-sec food reinforcement and extinction.

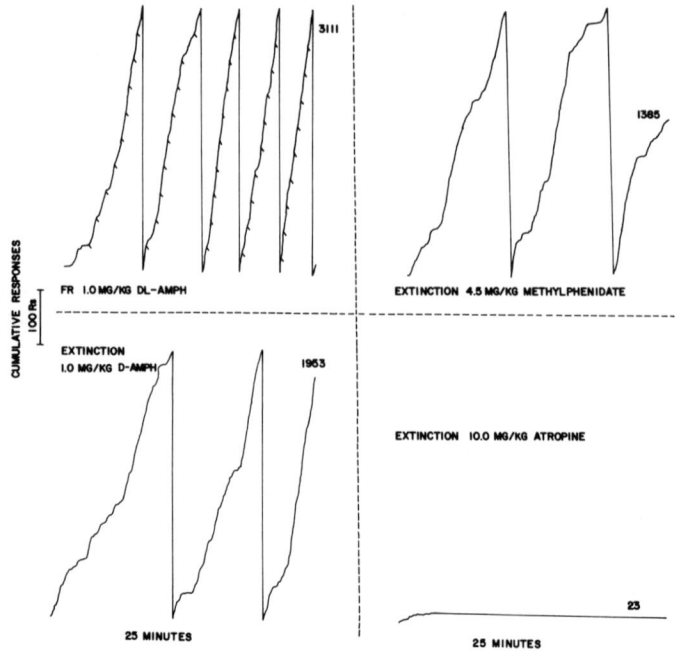

Fig. 11. Drug transfer. One-lever mult FR 50 EXT shock reinforcement and extinction.

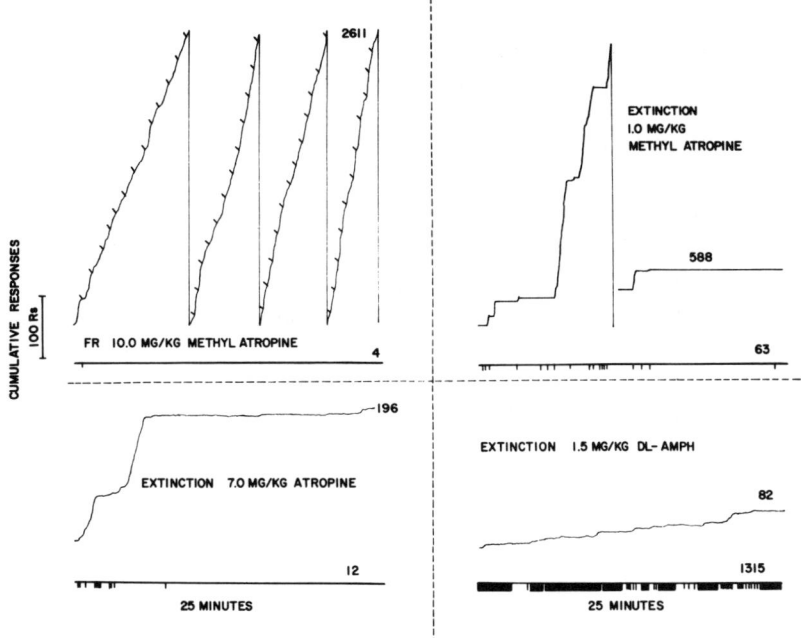

Fig. 12. Drug transfer. Two-lever mult FR 50 FR 50 shock reinforcement and extinction.

demonstrating a generalization of stimulus control for the three stimulant drugs. Under atropine (10.0 mg/kg), on the other hand, responding was suppressed, as had been the case during previous saline sessions, demonstrating the lack of transfer of control from dl-amphetamine to atropine.

Figure 12 presents a second case of drug generalization on a two-lever mult FR FR schedule in which methyl atropine (10.0 mg/kg) and saline (1.0 ml/kg were used as discriminative stimuli. FR responding on the methyl atropine lever is recorded cumulatively, and saline lever FR responding is recorded as marks of the event pen. Transfer of stimulus control from methyl atropine to atropine (7.0 mg/kg) occurred to a moderate degree. dl-Amphetamine (1.5 mg/kg) transferred to the saline lever, showing lack of generalization to methyl atropine.

While generalization of discriminative stimulus control between drugs within the same pharmacologic classification was readily obtained in these behavioral assays, it was also possible to bring responding under the discriminative control of such pairs of drugs, as shown with methyl atropine and atropine (compare Figure 5 with Figure 12). It is also interesting to note that subjects trained under atropine and saline when tested with methyl atropine show transfer to saline (data not presented graphically) which conflicts with the results shown in Figure 12. This can probably be explained by the fact that atropine mimics the peripheral effects of the quaternary form, but methyl atropine does not possess the CNS activity of atropine.

DISCRIMINATION REVERSAL

Figure 13 presents cumulative records of an animal trained on a two-lever mult FR 50 DRL 20-sec, with FR reinforcement under saline (1.0 mg/kg) and DRL reinforcement under *dl*-amphetamine (1.0 mg/kg), and then reversed to FR reinforcement under amphetamine and DRL under saline. The levers on which the schedules were programmed remained unchanged. The performance of the animal on the 20th day of reinforcement on the original and reversed contingencies is illustrative of the difficulty encountered in reversing the drug-schedule pairing. Under amphetamine, it was necessary to reduce the ratio requirement to 20 in order to obtain even brief periods of responding at a high rate. Responding during FR reinforcement under amphetamine remained sporadic throughout the 50 days of reversal training. The FR reinforcement session under amphetamine (shown in Figure 13) represents a special case in which the injection was made just

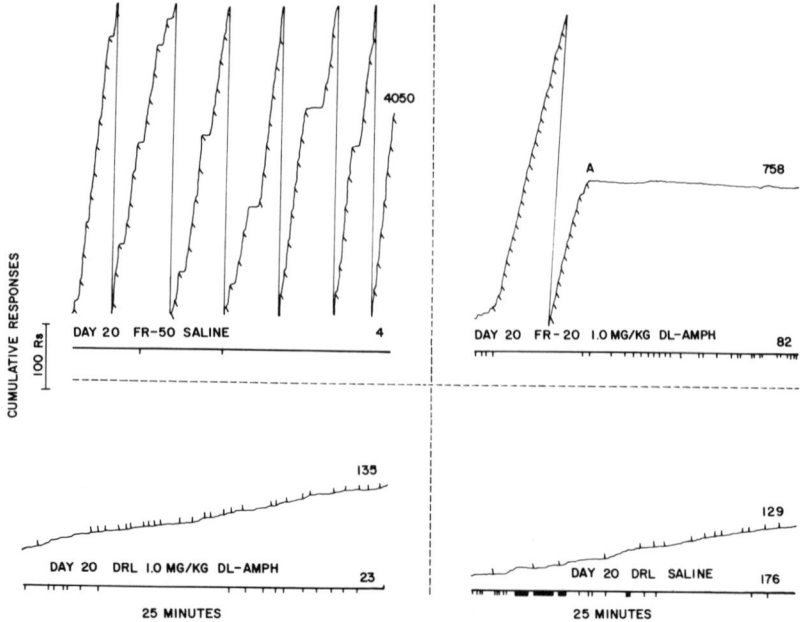

Fig. 13. Discrimination reversal. Two-lever mult FR 50 DRL 20-sec food reinforcement.

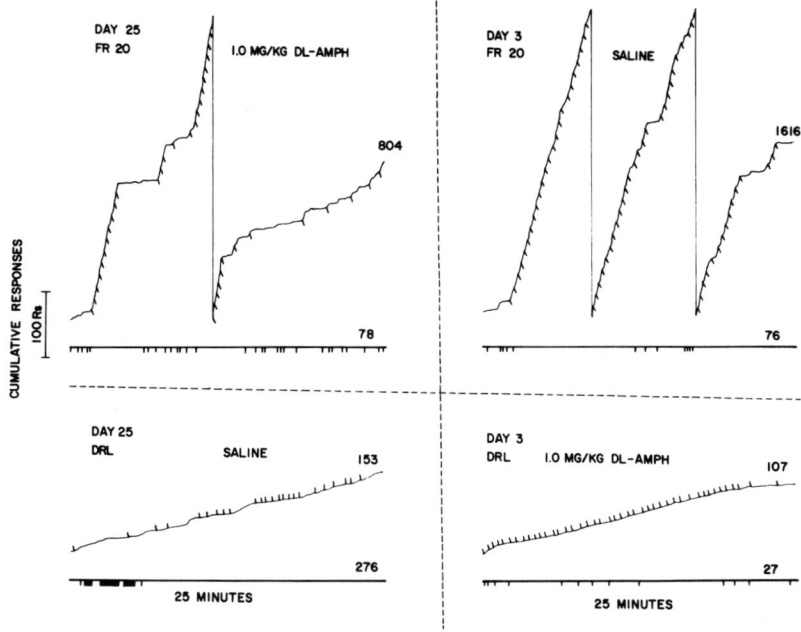

Fig. 14. Discrimination re-reversal. Two-lever mult FR 50 DRL 20-sec food reinforcement and extinction.

prior to the session rather than 15 minutes before. For the first 10 minutes, responding was at the high rate characteristic of FR reinforcement; but, from that point (A) to the end of the session the animal switched to the other lever and responded at a rate characteristic of DRL reinforcement. This switch probably coincided with the onset of the drug effect. Under saline, after reversal, the animal developed a fairly accurate rate on the DRL lever; however, bursts of responses on the FR lever occurred regularly during the initial 10 minutes of the session.

Extinction sessions, occasionally programmed during the period of reversal training (data not shown graphically), revealed discriminative control indicative of the pre-reversal drug-schedule contingencies.

Following 50 days of reinforcement under the reversal condition, the original drug-schedule pairing was reinstated. Figure 14 shows the last day of reversal training (left panels) and the third day of reversal for each component (right panels). Responding under both drug states was considerably more accurate under the reinstated condition than the reversal. In this sense, drugs function similarly to external stimuli (Ferster and Skinner, 1957) in that the control of responding is rapidly reinstated following re-reversal of the stimulus conditions.

These results suggest that behavior brought under drug control is difficult to alter. The relevance of these findings to problems of drug addiction has been discussed by the present authors elsewhere (Harris and Balster, 1969).

DRUG PROBES

Following 76 hours of training on a two-lever mult FR 50 DRL 20-sec schedule with *dl*-amphetamine (1.0 mg/kg) as the discriminative stimulus for DRL reinforcement and saline (1.0 mg/kg) as the discriminative stimulus for FR reinforcement, the schedule was changed to a two-lever mix FR 50 VI 30-sec schedule, and saline was administered prior to all sessions. The FR component was programmed on the originally paired lever, but VI reinforcement was programmed on the former DRL lever. Following 50 hours of training, extinction was initiated and an amphetamine "probe" injection given. Figure 15 shows the results of this procedure. The upper left panel shows the last day of responding on the DRL lever prior to VI training. The upper right panel shows extinction following DRL reinforcement. The lower left panel shows the last day of VI reinforcement. VI reinforcement produced a high rate of responding, predominantly on the lever programmed for VI reinforcement.

The lower right panel presents an extinction record when amphetamine was again administered. Responding occurred at a low steady rate characteristic of DRL reinforcement and primarily on the lever which had previously been associated with reinforcement under amphetamine.

Other drugs were substituted for amphetamine in further extinction tests with results agreeing closely with those found earlier in which methylphenidate and *d*-amphetamine simulated the discriminative-stimulus effects of *dl*-amphetamine, but other classes of drugs did not (data not presented graphically).

These data suggest that the passage of time, in and of itself, does not diminish the stimulus control of a drug. Further, they indicate that a period of interpolated training under a different drug state in the same experimental environment does not counteract the original control exercised by a drug over a particular form of behavior in that environment.

The practice of repeatedly using the same animals in different drug related experiments may be brought into question, particularly when the

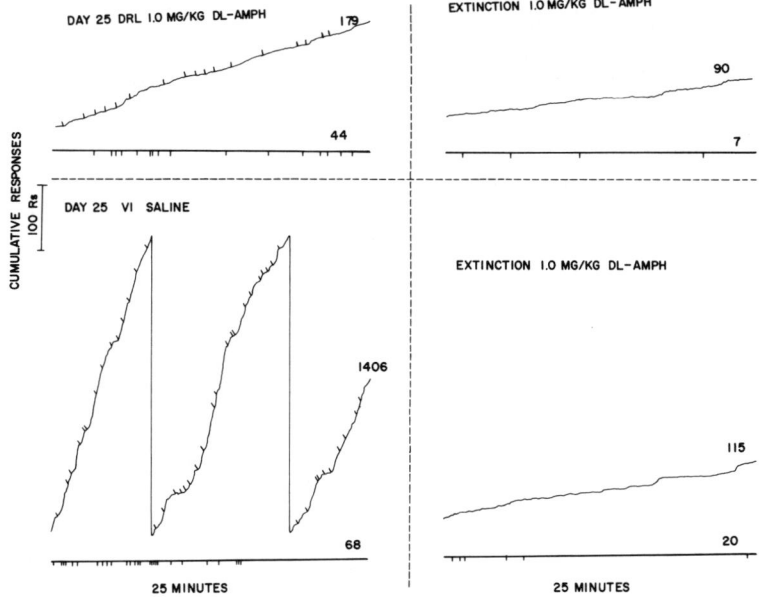

Fig. 15. Drug probe. Two-lever mult FR 50 DRL 20-sec food reinforcement and extinction.

animals have experienced drugs in contexts in which the drugs may have acquired stimulus control functions.

REFERENCES

Barry, H., Koepfer, E., and Lutch, J. Learning to discriminate between alcohol and nondrug condition. *Psychol. Rep.*, 1965, *16*, 1072.
—— and Kubena, R.K. An operant technique for learning discrimination between drug and nondrug state. Paper presented at American Psychological Association, Washington, D.C., September, 1967.
Bindra, D., Nyman, K., and Wise, J. Barbiturate-induced dissociation of acquisition and extinction: Role of movement-initiation processes. *J. Comp. Physiol. Psychol.*, 1965, *60*, 223.
Ferster, C.B., and Skinner, B.F. *Schedules of Reinforcement*, New York, Appleton-Century-Crofts, 1957.
Harris, R.T., and Balster, R.L. Discriminative control by *dl*-amphetamine and saline of lever choice and response patterning. *Psychonomic Science*, 1968, *10*, 109.
—— and Balster, R.L. An analysis of psychological dependence. In Harris, R.T., McIsaac, W.M., and Schuster, C.R., eds., *Advances in Mental Science: Drug Dependence*. Austin, University of Texas Press, 1969.

Heistad, G.T., and Torres, A.A. A mechanism for the effect of a tranquilizing drug on learned emotional responses. *University of Minnesota Medical Bulletin*, 1959, *30*, 518.

Korman, M., Knopf, I.J., and Leon, R.L. Alcohol as a discriminative stimulus: A preliminary report. *Texas Rep. Biol. Med.*, 1962, *20*, 61.

Overton, D.A. State-dependent or "dissociated" learning produced with pentobarbital. *J. Comp. Physiol. Psychol.*, 1964, *57*, 3.

—— State-dependent learning produced by depressant and atropine-like drugs. *Psychopharmacologia*, 1966, *10*, 6.

—— Dissociated learning in drug states (state-dependent learning). In *Psychopharmacology, A Review of Progress*. Washington: Public Health Service Publication No. 1836, 1968.

The Discriminate Control of a Food-Reinforced Operant by Interoceptive Stimulation[1]

Charles R. Schuster* and Joseph V. Brady**

*Department of Psychiatry,
University of Chicago,
Chicago, Illinois
**Division of Behavioral Biology
The Johns Hopkins University,
Baltimore, Maryland

In 1928 Bykov and Ivanova provided the first demonstration that interoceptive stimulation could become a conditioned stimulus in a classical conditioning paradigm (Bykov, 1957). Utilizing the classical conditioning technique, Bykov and his co-workers have subsequently demonstrated the existence of interoceptors in a wide variety of organs and tissues in the body. The extent of general scientific interest in this area is indicated by the fact that Bykov's major report of his thirty-year program on interoception has been translated into more foreign languages than any other Russian book in the field of medicine or biology (Razran, 1961).

The role of interoceptors in the control of operant behavior has unfortunately received only limited experimental attention. That operants may be brought under the stimulus control of interoceptors has been strongly suggested by the numerous studies requiring subjects to differentially respond on the basis of inferred physiologic changes induced by such manipulations as drug administration, or deprivation of food or water (Amsel, 1949; Conger, 1951; Heistad, 1957; Hull, 1933; Kendler, 1946; Leeper, 1935). Cook, Davidson, Davis, and Kelleher (1960) have demonstrated that avoid-

[1] The research reported in this chapter represents part of a dissertation submitted by the senior author to the Maryland University Graduate School in partial fulfillment of the requirements for the Ph.D. degree. This research was supported by research grant MY-1604 from the National Institute for Mental Health. The research reported here has previously been reported in the *Pavlov Journal of Higher Nervous Activity* (May-June, 1964, *14*, 448), which is published in Russian.

ance responses can be brought under the stimulus control of physiologic changes associated with the intravenous administration of epinephrine, norepinephrine, and acetylcholine, or the inflation of a balloon within a Thiry-Vella loop. More recently, Slucki, Adam, and Porter (1965) have shown that fixed-ratio responding for food reinforcement could be brought under the discriminative control of the interoceptive stimulation produced by inflation of a balloon in an isolated intestinal pouch.

The present investigation was concerned with demonstrating whether a food-reinforced operant could be brought under the discriminative control of interoceptive stimulation induced by (1) the intravenous infusion of epinephrine, and (2) the intravenous infusion of a saline-dextrose mixture into the superior vena cava. In addition to determining the existence of receptors in the superior vena cava, manipulations were carried out to define their characteristics and sensitivity.

GENERAL METHOD

Subjects and apparatus. The subjects in this investigation were four adult male rhesus monkeys selected from a stock colony on the basis of health and size. All subjects weighed between 4.0 and 6.0 kilograms and prior to this investigation were experimentally naive. Each animal was surgically prepared with a chronic polyethylene tubing catheter introduced into the internal jugular and terminating in the superior vena cava. The tubing was run subcutaneously to a midpoint on the animal's skull, where it was fixed in a skull-mounted bolt. Details of the surgical procedure are described elsewhere (Schuster, 1962).

The subjects were restrained in standard Foringer Primate Chairs to which were attached a lever manipulandum, a food pellet magazine, and a visual stimulus display panel. To prevent the animal from dislocating the catheter, the hand-hold covers on the restraining chair were kept closed. This necessitated utilization of a special mouth feeder in order to automatically dispense pellets of food to the subject. A cable, led through the wall, connected this equipment to a relay rack situated in an adjacent room. Stimulus presentations, food reinforcements, and recording of the subject's lever responses were accomplished automatically by means of electrical timers, counters, running time meters, stepping switches, and associated relay circuitry. Cumulative records were obtained using a Gerbrands Model C Cumulative Recorder.

The subjects were housed individually in a room 8 by 8 by 10 feet, with the back of the primate chair situated approximately 6 inches from the side wall. A 6-foot length of sterile polyethylene tubing (PE 100) was fixed with a needle juncture to the implanted catheter. This tubing was next run through a rubber stopper in the wall behind the chair. The tubing was fixed in the stopper with epoxy resin glue. White noise was on continuously in the experimental room to mask noises made by the experimenter and associated mechanical and electrical apparatus.

Procedure. The general procedure followed in this series of experiments was to bring a food-reinforced lever-pressing operant under the discriminative control of an interoceptive stimulus. A precise description of the nature of the interoceptive stimulation will be given in connection with each experiment. At the start of each experimental session the subjects had been deprived of food for approximately eighteen hours. Whenever possible, the subjects received their total daily food ration in the experimental session. In instances where this was not possible, the animals received the remainder of their daily food ration at the end of the experimental session. Water was available continuously.

A white light in the visual display panel was illuminated during each experimental session. During Session 1, the subjects were magazine trained to catch the pellets from the special mouth feeder. On a variable time schedule, with an average of four minutes, food pellets were automatically presented in the mouth feeder. The animals' ability to obtain these pellets was monitored by the experimenter. All the subjects were observed to obtain and eat the food pellets in the first four-hour session. The sound of the electric motor in the food magazine accompanied the presentation of the food pellets. A total of 60 food pellets were given to each subject in this session.

The subjects were given access to the lever manipulandum for the first time during Session 2. In the presence of the white house light each lever response was reinforced with the presentation of a single pellet of food. All subjects were conditioned to emit this response and received a total of 75 reinforcements within a two-hour experimental session.

In both experiments, discrimination training was initiated in Session 3. The details of the exact procedure will be described in conjunction with each of the experiments.

EXPERIMENT I

Method. Two subjects, surgically prepared and lever trained as previously described, were used in this experiment. Interoceptive stimulation was produced by infusion of an epinephrine solution through the chronic indwelling jugular catheter. The infusion sequence was as follows: (1) In the presence of the white house light a 60-second infusion period was intermittently presented. (2) In the first 20 seconds of the infusion period the animal was infused with 0.20 ml of the epinephrine solution. In this volume 20 mcg/kg of the drug was dissolved. (3) In the next 10 seconds the experimenter changed syringes to one containing 0.9 percent saline. (4) In the last 30 seconds of the infusion period 0.40 ml of saline was forced through the catheter in order to wash all the epinephrine solution into the subject. The above procedure will hereafter be referred to as an epinephrine trial.

Control infusion trials were carried out in the same manner as that described above with the exception that in Step 2, 0.9 percent saline was used rather than the epinephrine solution. This will hereafter be referred to as a saline control trial.

Injections were made manually from 1-ml tuberculin syringes by the experimenter. The rate of infusion was held constant by careful attention to a wall clock with a sweep second hand. Every attempt was made to keep the injection procedure constant for both the epinephrine and saline control trials. In each daily session a total of 25 epinephrine trials were randomly alternated with 25 saline control trials. All trials were presented on a variable time schedule with a minimum of 120 and a maximum of 480 seconds. A response, separating each trial, occurring within 60 seconds after the termination of the epinephrine trial was reinforced with three pellets of food. Responses in the 60-second interval following the saline control infusion sequence were never reinforced with food. Table 1 gives the procedure followed in the discrimination training.

Beginning with Session 11 the number of responses required for delivery of the food reinforcement was increased to five (FR 5). Following Sessions 18 and 27 the dosage of epinephrine was decreased. This was done because of certain undesirable side effects produced by the drug. At the higher dosages the subjects periodically showed vomiting in close temporal contiguity with the drug administration. The number of responses made in the 60-second interval following epinephrine and saline infusions were recorded for each presentation. This was converted to a percentage of times that the subject met the ratio requirement in saline and epinephrine trials in each daily session.

Results. Figure 1 shows the percentage of saline control and epinephrine trials in which the subjects met the fixed-ratio requirement. In Sessions 3 to 10 this percentage showed a gradual increase for both the epinephrine and saline control trials. When the response requirement was increased to FR 5 in Session 11 this percentage showed a slight decline. In subsequent sessions, however, the percentage continued to increase. By

Table 1. *Discrimination training procedure*

Session	Epinephrine Dosage mcg/kg	No. of Epinephrine Trials	No. of Saline Control Trials	No. of Responses Required for Reinforcement
3-4	20	25	25	1
5-10	20	25	25	1
11-17	20	25	25	5
18-27*	15	25	25	5
28-57	10	25	25	5

* E^1 only following Session 27.

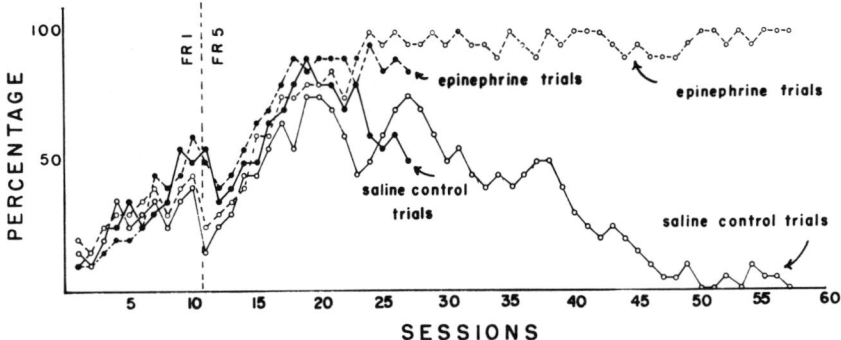

Fig. 1. Percentage of epinephrine and saline control trials in which the subject met the response requirements for reinforcement.

Session 18 the subjects met the fixed-ratio requirement more than 75 percent of the time. There was, however, no difference between the non-reinforced saline control trials and the reinforced epinephrine trials. Evidence of differential stimulus control by the epinephrine infusion was not observed until Session 23. Beginning with Session 23 the subjects showed a gradual decrement in emitting the fixed-ratio of five responses in the saline control trials.

Subject E-2 died following Session 27. The remaining results were obtained from Subject E-1 only.

For Subject E-1 the epinephrine infusion has clearly gained discriminative control over the lever-pressing operant by Session 47. In Sessions 47 to 57 the subject rarely responded following the saline control infusion whereas the subject met the ratio requirement almost 100 percent of the time following the epinephrine administration. Following Session 57 Subject E-1 died.

Discussion. The demonstration that a food-reinforced operant can be brought under the discriminative control of interoceptive changes produced by the administration of epinephrine is a logical extension of prior reports.

As previously reviewed, Cook et al. (1960) have demonstrated that avoidance responding in dogs can be brought under the stimulus control of intravenous administration of epinephrine. The present findings confirm this earlier investigation in showing that drug-induced interoceptive changes can act as a discriminative stimulus for a food-reinforced operant.

The most striking result obtained in the present investigation is that the lever-pressing operant came under the discriminative control of the infusion of both epinephrine and saline. This is indicated by the increased frequency of responding for both types of trials in the first 15 to 20 sessions. Presumably the subjects are showing generalization from the reinforced epinephrine infusions to the non-reinforced saline infusions. The results suggest that the infusion of saline through the jugular catheter into the superior vena cava was discriminable to the subjects. Because of this unexpected finding, a second experiment was undertaken to specify the conditions under which a monkey's operant behavior could be brought under the discriminative control of this infusion procedure.

EXPERIMENT II

Methods. Two subjects (DM 2 and DM 3), surgically prepared and lever trained as previously described, were used in the experiment.

Interoceptive stimulation was produced by infusing a 5 percent dextrose-saline solution into the superior vena cava at a rate of 2.00 ml/min. These S^D infusion periods were controlled by a Harvard Infusion Apparatus (Model No. 410) modified so that infusion periods could be intermittently programmed. Control infusion periods consisted of the infusion of the dextrose-saline mixture at a rate of 0.04 ml/min. The rate of infusion for the control and S^D infusion periods was manually preset by the experimenter using the dial adjustment on the Harvard Infusion Apparatus.

The S^D and control infusion periods continued at each presentation until the subject emitted a lever pressing response or until 30 seconds had elapsed. A response during the S^D infusion period had two consequences: (1) the infusion was terminated, and (2) a reinforcement of two food pellets was delivered to the subject. Responses during the control infusion periods also had two consequences: (1) the termination of the infusion, and (2) the occurrence of a two-minute "time-out" period during which all experimental stimuli and the timer controlling infusion period presentations were turned off. The number of responses required for the above mentioned consequences was increased in Sessions 4 to 8 from 1 to 10. This will be referred to as a fixed ratio of ten responses or FR 10.

Each daily experimental session lasted for approximately five hours. A white light in the visual display was illuminated during the experimental session except during time-out periods. In the course of the five-hour session, 50 S^D infusion and 50 control infusion periods were randomly presented on a variable time schedule. A minimum of 60 and a maximum of 300 seconds separated each infusion presentation.

Latency measures from the onset of the infusion period to the emission of the tenth response, were separately recorded in 0.01 of a minute for S^D and control infusion periods. In addition, the frequency of S^D and control infusion periods in which the fixed ratio of ten responses occurred was recorded and converted into percentages for each experimental session. Cumulative records of each daily session were obtained.

Following stabilization of the subject's behavior, the rate of infusion was varied systematically over five values: 0.125, 0.25, 0.50, 1.00 and 2.00 ml/min. Emission of ten responses during the 30-second infusion period at all values was reinforced with a single food pellet. In Sessions 46 to 55 each subject was given 100 S^D infusion presentations at each of these values to allow stabilization of their performance. During the next ten sessions (56 to 65) the five infusion rates were presented systematically. In each daily session 10 S^D infusion periods were given at each rate. Ten control infusion periods were also presented daily. The sequence of presentation was randomized immediately prior to each daily session.

Latency measures, from the onset of the infusion period to the time taken for the subjects to emit ten responses, were separately recorded in units of 0.01 of a minute for all the infusion rates. The frequency of meeting the FR 10 requirement was also separately recorded for all infusion rates.

Results. After approximately 35 sessions, the lever-pressing operant of both subjects was seen to be under the discriminative control of the S^D infusion periods. Figure 2 shows a 1-hour sample cumulative record taken from Session 39 for both subjects. This record shows that the subjects consistently emitted the FR 10 in the S^D infusion periods. In contrast the animals rarely responded as frequently as ten times in the 30-second control infusion period. Table 2 shows the percentages for both subjects in Sessions 41 to 45. The subjects met the FR 10 requirement over 90 percent of the time in the S^D infusion periods while the percentage of control trials in which the subjects emitted ten responses was consistently below 35 percent.

Table 3 shows the average latencies from the same sessions in 0.01 of a minute from the onset of the S^D and control infusion periods to the occurrence of the tenth response. The consistent and marked difference in the latencies between the control and S^D infusion periods reflects the degree of stimulus control exercised by the S^D infusion procedure.

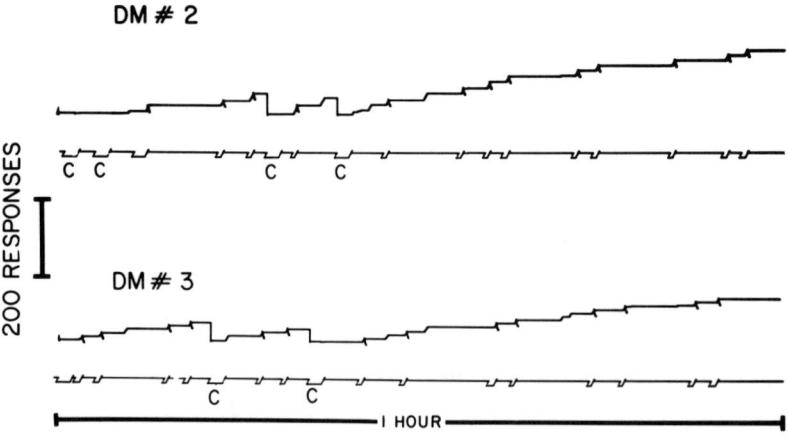

Fig. 2. Representative cumulative records under baseline performance conditions. C=Control infusion periods.

Table 2. Percentage of S^D and control infusion periods in which subjects emitted ten responses

	Subjects DM #2		Subjects DM #3	
Session No.	% S^D Infusion	% Control Infusion	% S^D Infusion	% Control Infusion
41	96	20	100	32
42	100	32	92	24
43	92	32	96	20
44	100	24	100	32
45	100	28	96	32

Table 3. Average latencies in 0.01 of a minute from S^D or control infusion onset to emission of the tenth response

	Subject DM #2		Subject DM #3	
Session No.	S^D Infusion Latencies	Control Infusion Latencies	S^D Infusion Latencies	Control Infusion Latencies
41	.13	.46	.11	.42
42	.10	.42	.10	.40
43	.11	.44	.13	.41
44	.09	.39	.12	.45
45	.13	.42	.11	.40

Since the latency measure and the percentage of trials in which the subjects met the FR 10 requirement were found to be stable over Sessions 41 to 45, parametric investigation of discriminative control of operant behavior as a function of infusion rate was started in Session 46.

Figure 3 shows the percentage of trials in which the subjects met the FR

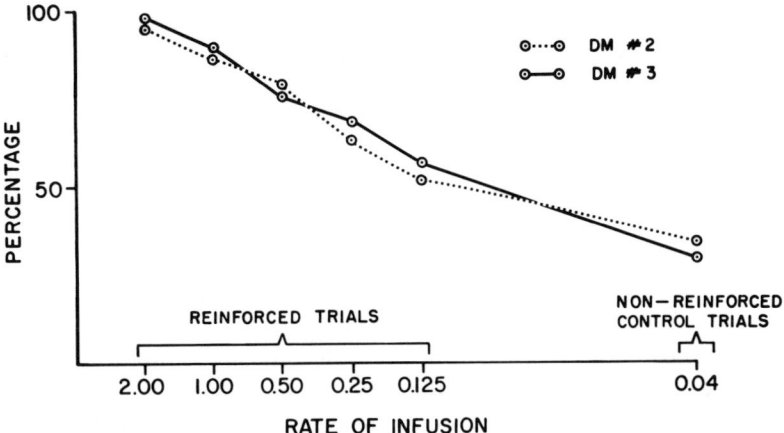

Fig. 3. Percentage of trials in which subjects met Fixed Ratio 10 requirement as a function of rate of infusion. Each point represents 100 trials.

10 requirement as a function of the five S^D infusion rates and control infusions. At the highest infusion rate of 2.00 ml/min both subjects met the FR 10 requirement over 90 percent of the time.

The percentage of trials in which the subjects met the FR 10 requirement varied directly as a function of infusion rate. At the lower infusion rates of 0.25 to 0.125 ml/min the percentage approximated that obtained in the non-reinforced control infusion periods.

Figure 4 illustrates changes in latencies to the tenth response as a

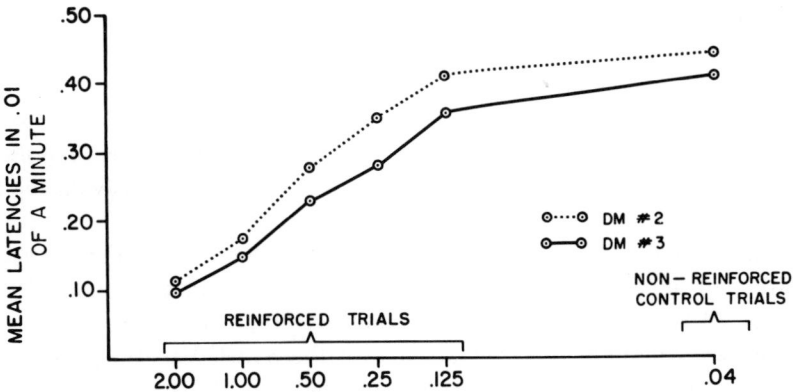

Fig. 4. Latencies from onset of infusion S^D to emission of tenth response as a function of rate of infusion. Each point represents mean of 100 trials.

function of the rate of infusion. As the rate of infusion decreased, latencies to the tenth response showed a consistent increment. At the lowest infusion rates of 0.25 and 0.125 ml/min the latencies for both subjects approximated those obtained for the non-reinforced control infusion periods.

Discussion. The results of this experiment demonstrated that an operant can be brought under the control of the infusion of a dextrose-saline mixture into the superior vena cava. From the parametric study of infusion rates it can be stated that rates at least as low as 0.50 ml/min can acquire significant discriminative control over the lever-pressing operant. These conclusions were based on the observed differences in the subject's performance in the S^D infusion periods and the control infusion periods. Before concluding that the discrimination was based upon differential interoceptive stimulation, however, it is necessary to rule out any possible differential exteroceptive cues associated with the different infusion rates. The two most likely sources of exteroceptive stimulation were those associated with temperature of the infused solution and with vibrations of the catheter induced by the Harvard Infusion Apparatus. Control studies were therefore performed to assess the role of such factors in determining the results of this experiment.

CONTROL STUDIES FOR EXPERIMENT II

Vibration. Following Experiment II, Subjects DM 2 and DM 3 were returned to the baseline condition in which the S^D infusion rate was fixed at 2.00 ml/min. For five consecutive sessions 50 S^D and 50 control infusion periods were given daily. Latencies from the onset of the infusion periods to the completion of the tenth response were recorded separately. The frequency of meeting the FR 10 requirement under the different conditions were also recorded separately.

In Session 71, the polyethylene catheter was firmly taped to a 3-inch, 8-ohm Varsity speaker at a distance of 15 inches above the insertion point of the tubing into the subject. The speaker was driven continuously during this session by a Foringer White Noise Generator.

Figure 5 shows the percentage of times that the subjects met the FR 10 requirement in the S^D infusion periods in Sessions 70, 71, and 72. In Sessions 70 and 72 the baseline procedure was followed. In Session 71 the catheter was vibrated by being taped over the 3-inch Varsity speaker. The percentage of trials in which the subjects met the FR 10 requirement was not significantly affected by the addition of the vibration to the catheter. The ineffectiveness of this vibratory procedure to mask the infusion S^D is

The Discriminate Control of a Food-Reinforced Operant   143

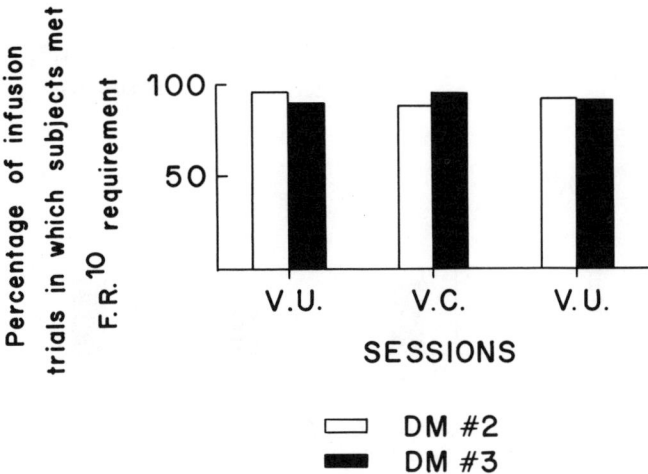

Fig. 5. Percentage of trials (N=50) in which subjects met FR 10 requirement in sessions with (V.C.) and without (V.U.) vibration of catheter.

further shown by the latency data in Figure 6. The latencies in Sessions 70 and 72 were not significantly different from those obtained in Session 71.

Figure 7 reveals an especially pertinent fact. In Session 71, where the catheter was purposely vibrated, the percentage of control trials in which the subjects emitted ten responses was consistently below that seen in Sessions 70 and 72.

Thermal. In Session 74 the saline-dextrose mixture was heated to a temperature of 100 degrees Fahrenheit at the point of entry of the catheter into the subject.

Figure 8 shows the percentage of time that the subject met the FR 10

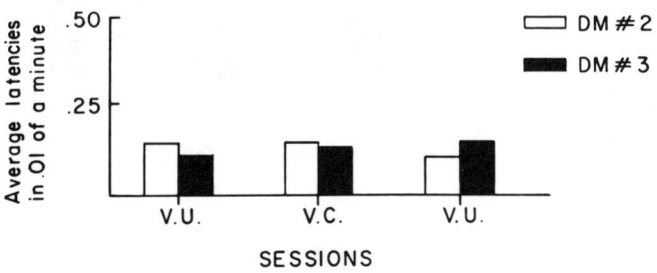

Fig. 6. Latencies to the tenth response in infusion S^D in sessions with (V.C.) and without (V.U.) vibration of catheter.

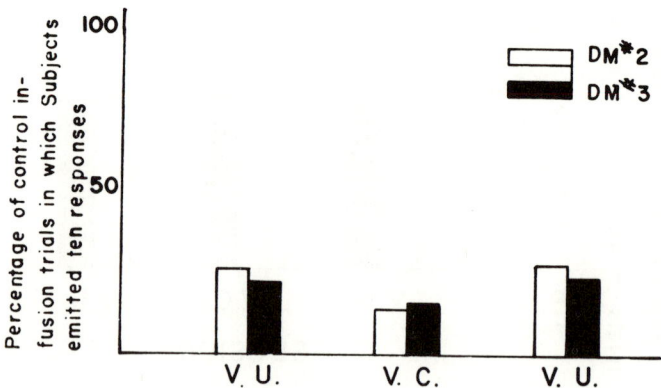

Fig. 7. Percentage of control trials (N=50) in which subjects emitted ten responses in sessions with (V.C.) and without (V.U.) vibration of catheter.

requirement in the S^D infusion periods in Sessions 73, 74, and 75. In Sessions 73 and 75 the temperature of the infused solution was uncontrolled to the extent that room temperature fluctuations occurred. In Session 74 the solution reached the subject at a temperature of approximately 100 to 102 degrees Fahrenheit. The manipulation produced no change in the frequency with which the subjects met the FR 10 requirement in the S^D infusion periods. The failure of this manipulation to alter the subjects' discrimination

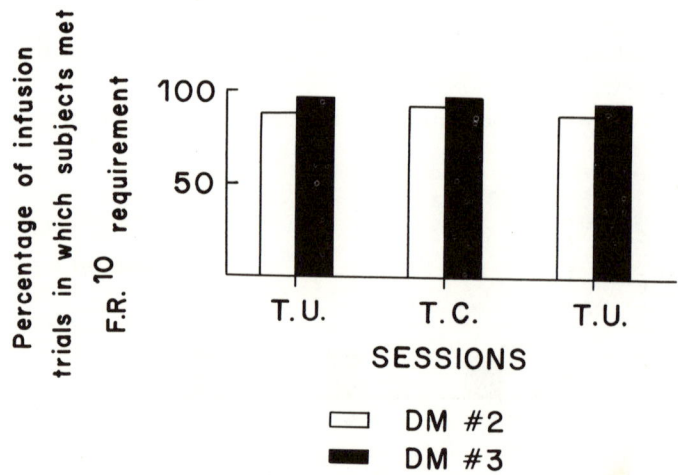

Fig. 8. Percentage of trials (N=50) in which subjects met FR 10 requirement when infusion temperature was uncontrolled (T.U.) and when heated to 100°F (T.C.).

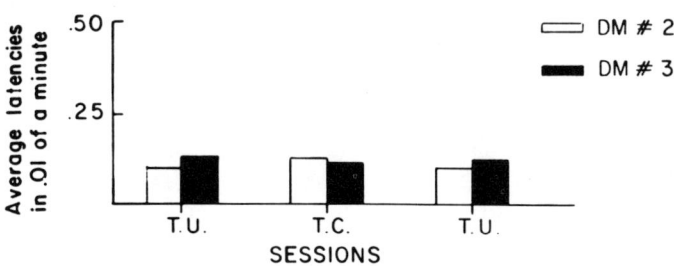

Fig. 9. Latencies to the tenth response in infusion S^D when infusion temperature was uncontrolled (T.U.) and when heated to 100°F (T.C.).

is also reflected by the latency data given in Figure 9. The latencies shown here for sessions without the temperature control was not significantly different from the sessions where the solution was heated to approximately 100 degrees Fahrenheit.

Chemical constituents. In Sessions 76, 77, and 78 the infused solution was systematically varied from 0.9 percent saline-5 percent dextrose mixture to either 5 percent dextrose in sterile water or 0.9 percent saline. Blocks of six S^D infusions using each of the three solutions were randomly presented over the course of these three sessions. The subjects were reinforced for emitting the FR 10 in all of the S^D infusion periods regardless of the constituents of the solution. Since it was impossible to drain the catheter connection to the subject, the data from the first S^D infusion period following a change in solution were discounted. This trial served essentially to refill the cather with the new solution being tested. This gave a total of 50

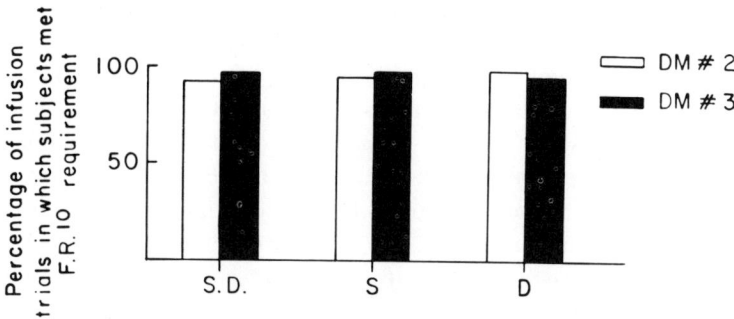

Fig. 10. Percentage of trials (N=50) in which subjects met FR 10 requirement as a function of the chemical constituents of the infusion S^D.

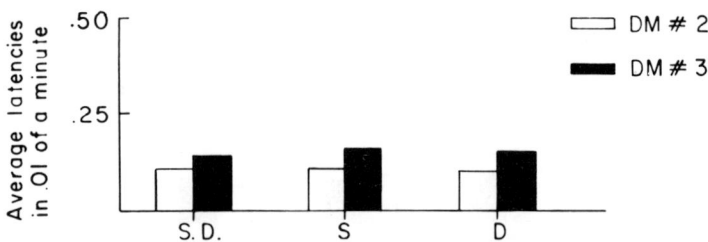

Fig. 11. Latencies to the tenth response in infusion S^D as a function of the chemical constituents of the infusion.

S^D infusion periods with each of the three solutions from which the subjects' performance was recorded.

Figure 10 shows the percentage of trials in which the subjects met the FR 10 requirement in S^D infusion periods as a function of the three types of solution: (1) 0.9 percent saline-5 percent dextrose, (2) 0.9 percent saline, and (3) 5 percent dextrose in sterile water. These results failed to reflect any differences in the stimulus control in the infusion S^D as a function of the different constituents in the solution. The latency measures, shown in Figure 11, also failed to reflect any change in the discriminative control of the infusion procedures as a function of the different chemical constituents.

GENERAL DISCUSSION

The control studies in the previous section failed to give any evidence that the discriminative control exerted by the S^D infusion procedure was based upon thermal or vibratory stimulation. It seems likely, however, that vibratory stimulation common to both S^D and control infusion periods may account for the subjects responding periodically in the control infusion periods. The decrement seen in the frequency of responding in the control infusion periods when the catheter was continuously vibrated may have been caused by the "masking" of the vibratory cues induced by energizing the Harvard Infusion Apparatus. The fact that the stimulus control exerted by the infusion S^D was not disrupted by the continuous vibration of the catheter indicated, however, that the vibratory stimulation caused by the Harvard Infusion Apparatus was not a necessary condition for the discrimination. The procedure of continuously vibrating the catheter may be found useful in future research for "masking" potential sources of vibratory stimulation.

On the basis of the evidence obtained in the control studies it may be concluded that the discriminative control exerted by the infusion of the saline-dextrose solution into the superior vena cava was based upon the stimulation of interoceptors. The exact nature and location of these interoceptors cannot as yet be specified, since the data in this report suggest only certain logical possibilities.

The fact that the discriminative control exerted by the S^D infusion procedure was comparably effective when the infused solution was changed from dextrose-saline to 0.9 percent saline indicated that neither systemic or local effects of the dextrose were necessary conditions for this discrimination. The comparable stimulus control exerted by the infusion of the 5 percent dextrose in sterile water also ruled out systemic or local effects of the NaCl as the basis of this discrimination.

The existence of baroreceptors in the circulatory system has been demonstrated (Bykov, 1957) and suggests the possibility that such receptors located in the superior vena cava could be involved in the present discrimination. This possibility seems unlikely, however, since rates of infusion as low as 0.50 ml/min were found to exert significant discriminative control over the subjects' behavior. The average volume of the dextrose-saline mixture which the subjects received in each S^D infusion period at the rate of 0.50 ml/min was less than 0.40 ml. In the same period as this infusion approximately 300 to 400 ml of venous blood was returned into the superior vena cava (Nieman, Schuster, and Thompson, 1962). Normal fluctuations in the volume of venous blood returning through the superior vena cava are far greater than that produced by the infusion procedure, and it would be difficult to conceive how the baroreceptors could serve as the basis for the observed discrimination under these conditions.

The results of the thermal control study, in which the dextrose-saline solution was heated to approximately the subjects' body temperature, would seem to rule out thermal receptors in any location as the basis of this discrimination. Further, the warming of the dextrose-saline mixture by the blood in the superior vena cava would be extremely rapid because of the volume differences involved.

Several experimental manipulations remain to be explored in future investigations in an effort to specify the exact nature of the stimulus and interoceptors involved in this discrimination. A technique is currently being developed which will allow the use of the subject's own venous blood as the infused solution. The physical and chemical properties of the withdrawn blood will be maintained unchanged. If the infusion of blood can be shown to gain discriminative control over the lever pressing operant then chemoreceptors can be excluded as the possible neural basis of this discrimination.

Both Experiments I and II demonstrate that a food-reinforced operant can be brought under the discriminative control of interoceptive stimulation. This fact has both methodological and theoretical implications. First, the use of the operant paradigm for establishing discrimination has been shown applicable to investigating the existence and sensitivity of at least certain types of interoceptors. Neurophysiologists, psychopharmacologists, as well as psychologists may find this a valuable procedure for establishing a behavioral baseline for studing changes in the sensitivity of interoceptors as a function of experimental manipulations appropriate to these disciplines. Future research will determine the relative efficacy of this procedure, as compared to the classical conditioning paradigm, as a means of studying interoceptors. Hopefully, both methods can be used to confirm and extend important new facts relevant to the experimental analysis of behavior.

REFERENCES

Amsel, A. Selective association and the anticipatory goal response mechanism as explanatory concepts in learning theory. *J. Exp. Psychol.*, 1949, *39*, 785.

Bykov, K.M. *The Cerebral Cortex and the Internal Organs.* Translated and edited by W.H. Gantt. New York, Chemical Publishing Co., Inc., 1957.

Conger, J.J. The effects of alcohol on conflict behavior in the albino rat. *Quart. J. Stud. Alcohol*, 1951, *12*, 1.

Cook, L., Davidson, A., Davis, D.J., and Kelleher, R.T. Epinephrine, norepinephrine, and acetylcholine as conditioned stimuli for avoidance behavior. *Science*, 1960, *131*, 990.

Heistad, G.T. A biopsychological approach to somatic treatments in psychiatry. *Amer. J. Psychiat.*, 1957, *114*, 540.

Hull, C.L. Differential habituation to internal stimuli in the albino rat. *J. Comp. Psychol.*, 1933, *16*, 255.

Kendler, H.H. The influence of simultaneous hunger and thirst drives upon the learning or two opposed spatial responses of the white rat. *J. Exp. Psychol.*, 1946, *36*, 212.

Leeper, R. The role of motivation in learning: A study of the phenomenon of differential motivational control of the utilization of habits. *J. Genet. Psychol.*, 1935, *46*, 3.

Nieman, W.I., Schuster, R.C., and Thompson, T. A surgical preparation for chronic intravenous infusion in rhesus monkeys. Technical Report No. 6230, Laboratory of Psychopharmacology, The University of Maryland. 1962.

Razran, G. The observable unconscious and the inferable conscious in current Soviet psychophysiology: Interoceptive conditioning, semantic conditioning and the orienting reflex. *Psychol. Rev.*, 1961, *68*, 81.

Schuster, C.R. The discriminative control of operant behavior by interoceptive stimulation. Doctoral thesis, University of Maryland, 1962.

Slucki, H., Adam, G., and Porter, R.W. Operant discrimination of an interoceptive stimulus in rhesus monkeys. *J. Exp. Anal. Behav.*, 1965, *8*, 405.

Spector, W.S., ed. *Handbook of Biological Data.* Philadelphia, W.B. Saunders Company, 1956.

Discriminative Stimulus Functions of Drugs: Interpretations. I

A. Charles Catania

Department of Psychology
New York University
New York, New York

In any study of drugs, it is difficult if not impossible to ignore the fundamental pharmacologic principle that no drug has a single action. The principle is important not only because it is relevant to specific experimental problems but also because it so precisely parallels a principle of overriding importance in the analysis of behavior: no stimulus has a single action. We ordinarily speak of this behavioral principle in terms of the multiple functions of stimuli, and it is illustrated in any experiment concerned with controlling relationships between stimuli and responses. For example, an experiment that deals with an elicitation relationship must be designed carefully to avoid confounding elicitation with the potential reinforcing or discriminative effects of the eliciting stimulus. The principle is also illustrated in the organization of this book, which, in speaking of the stimulus properties of drugs, separates these into discriminative and eliciting and reinforcing properties.

The very similarity of the pharmacologic principle that no drug has a single action and the behavioral principle that no stimulus has a single action leads us to the conclusion that the treatment of drugs as stimuli must be fundamental to psychopharmacologic research. When we speak of the effects of drugs on behavior, we often lapse into such expressions as that the administration of a drug produces a stimulus the receptor for which has not been identified. But it is not appropriate to say that the drug *produces* a stimulus; rather, the drug *is* a stimulus. The most important difference between drugs and stimuli taken from the familiar sensory modalities is probably only in the route of administration. Nor do we have to identify a receptor before we can speak of a drug as a stimulus. Discriminative control involves a behavioral relationship, a relationship between environmental events and responses; once this relationship has been established, its behavioral status is not altered by demonstrating the involvement of a particular part of the anatomy.

Schuster and Brady's chapter (Chapter 8) deals with the resourceful but unsuccessful pursuit of the basis for a subtle interoceptive discrimination. Toward the end of their chapter, one is left almost with a feeling of awe about the subtlety with which the stimulus is discriminated. There is no denying the mystery and thus the challenge posed by discriminative performances such as these. Yet it is also important to note that the problems that exist with respect to what drugs do are not really different in principle from the problems that exist with respect to what any stimulus does.

Consider, for example, the role of temporal discrimination in the analysis of behavior. We may study such discriminations by reinforcing one response after a stimulus has been presented for one duration and a different response after the stimulus has been presented for another duration (e.g., in the rat, left-lever presses after two-second tones and right-lever presses after four-second tones). If responses come under the control of the temporal properties of the stimulus, the basis for the performance may seem almost mystical, in the sense that we do not know of any temporal receptor—we do not know of any place in the organism where time is discriminated or any organ through which temporal stimuli pass. Yet this does not prevent us from studying the functional properties of temporal discrimination; we can study its psychophysics (e.g., difference thresholds for duration) without knowing anything about the temporal receptor (Catania, 1970).

We therefore can proceed in one of two ways when we set about to study the discriminative effects of drugs. On the one hand, we can examine the functional properties of discriminative control; on the other, we can search for the mechanism of action or, in other words, for the drug receptor. In the first case, we establish a stimulus-control relationship between drugs and behavior and then, by administering different doses of the drugs or by administering different drugs, we explore the functional properties of this control: thresholds, the dimensions along which drugs are generalized, and interactions with behavioral contingencies such as the schedule of reinforcement or the temporal parameters of stimulus presentation. The endeavor differs from that in the second case, which is concerned with the mechanism of control, much as the study of the psychophysics of vision differs from the study of the biochemistry of visual pigments or the neurophysiology of the visual system. Once stimulus control has been demonstrated with a particular drug, the question of the receptor for that drug is not behavioral and therefore need not bear on a functional analysis of the drug's effects. We do not have to find a receptor to speak of drug function. This, of course, is not to say that we should not go about the search for the mechanism of drug control, but rather simply that we should recognize that these two different avenues are open to us. One leads to a functional and behavioral analysis of stimulus control, and the other leads to an anatomic, physiologic, or biochemical description of the effects of the stimulus.

We should also note that, though there are differences in emphasis, the methodologies of functional analysis in pharmacology and in behavior demonstrate their common foundations. Pharmacologists have taught psychologists to recognize that little can be learned about drugs on the basis of the administration of single doses. But the determination of dose-response functions, which is fundamental to pharmacologic analysis, is paralleled by the psychologist's variation of stimulus properties, which is essential to the determination of controlling dimensions of stimuli (e.g., as in studies of attention or generalization).

Drugs may well have characteristics that give stimulus control by some drugs unusual properties, but it does not follow that we should treat any drug as a variable of a different sort than other stimulus variables that we impose on behavior. It is sometimes tempting to assume that a difference in receptor mechanism implies a difference in the functional properties of stimulus control, but even a difference in behavioral outcomes does not force such an assumption. The detailed characteristics of drug control may differ no more from one drug to another or from drugs to other stimuli than the characteristics of stimulus control differ from one sensory modality to another. Many differences in stimulus control within the familiar sensory modalities (e.g., vision or hearing), as well as within modalities that are less easily specifiable (e.g., those of temporal discrimination), depend on idiosyncratic properties of the mode of stimulus delivery. For example, visual stimuli are ordinarily localized in an experimental environment in a different way than auditory stimuli, and temporal stimuli have in common with drugs the special characteristic that it takes time to present them, so that they cannot be varied discontinuously in the presence of an organism. It is therefore reassuring to see that, when researchers examine stimulus-control procedures involving drugs, they are more careful in these than in earlier times to match the parameters of their discriminative situations (e.g., temporal spacing of discriminative and reinforcing stimuli) to those of analogous situations involving control by more familiar exteroceptive stimuli.

The point is illustrated in Doctor Overton's analysis (Chapter 6) of the way in which dissociation phenomena might be treated as special instances of stimulus generalization. One concern was the asymmetry of dissociations.

But asymmetries are not unknown even in the more familiar sensory modalities. For example, stimulus-control procedures based on the intensive properties of stimuli (prothetic continua) are more likely to yield asymmetrical gradients than those based on non-intensive properties (metathetic continua). We would not expect generalization or post-discrimination gradients determined along the prothetic dimension of sound intensity to have the same properties as gradients determined along the metathetic dimension of sound frequency. The point is not that asymmetrical gradients obtained along intensive sensory continua should be taken as of the same sort or as having the same basis as asymmetries in stimulus control by drugs, but rather that the finding of asymmetrical outcomes when drugs function as discriminative stimuli need not be taken as an embarrassment to the analysis of drug effects in terms of stimulus control.

The problem of multiple functions of stimuli will inevitably arise in these areas of research (e.g., as when an asymmetrical gradient along an intensive continuum is treated as a summation of two effects, one involving discriminative control and the other, in the relationship called stimulus-intensity dynamism, involving elicitation). In fact, the problems are more serious with drug stimuli than with stimuli from more familiar modalities. We already know a good deal about the potential eliciting and reinforcing properties of the stimuli in modalities such as vision or audition, but when we explore the unfamiliar ground of drug stimuli we must be prepared to encounter novel interactions between the several stimulus functions. For example, in the chapter by Harris and Balster (Chapter 7), the discriminative effects of amphetamine were examined with different reinforcement schedules operating in the drugged and in the undrugged condition, and it was made evident that proper evaluation of the findings required not only an analysis of the quality of stimulus control but also an assessment of the direct and differential effects of amphetamine on behavior maintained by fixed-ratio and other schedules of reinforcement.

The difficulty we have in speaking consistently about drugs as stimuli may be compounded by the two different strategies that guide psychopharmacologic experiments. In administering drugs on a baseline of behavior, we can stress our interest in finding out something about behavior or our interest in finding out something about the drugs. We may be able to discriminate among behavioral processes by discovering drugs that differentially affect these processes, or we may be able to discriminate among classes of drugs by discovering differential effects on various behavioral processes. An example may illustrate both this distinction and the relevance of a concern with multiple function. The account that follows does not bear directly on discriminative control by drugs, but it shows how our preconceptions can distract us from specific and relatively simple stimulus properties of drugs.

A comparison of schedules of positive and negative reinforcement was the concern of experiments I conducted in collaboration with Doctor L. Cook at the Smith, Kline and French Laboratories. Our strategy was to superimpose drugs on schedules that were identical with respect to temporal parameters, properties of performance, and other features, except for the differential consequences: presentation of food or escape from shock. Data from a 10-minute fixed-interval schedule of food reinforcement that maintained lever pressing in the squirrel monkey were already available in the laboratory; we therefore established a 10-minute fixed-interval schedule of negative reinforcement, in which the lever press was reinforced by a period of escape from electric shock (details have been presented in Cook and Catania, 1964).

Drugs such as chlorpromazine, meprobamate, chlordiazepoxide, and amphetamine had effects on performances maintained by negative reinforcement that were comparable to their characteristic effects on performances maintained by positive reinforcement. The similarity of outcomes was consistent with our recognition that the distinction between positive and negative reinforcement is to some extent arbitrary (e.g., as when heat as a reinforcer for the lever presses of a rat in a cold environment may be interpreted either as positive reinforcement by the presentation of heat or negative reinforcement by escape from the cold).

But then came a surprising outcome. When appropriate doses of imipramine were administered on the fixed-interval escape performance, the reduction of responding typical with schedules of positive reinforcement was observed on the day of drug administration, but a reliable elevation of responding above the baseline level was observed 24 hours later. This effect had not been observed with the corresponding schedules of positive reinforcement. Here was a finding with potential relevance both for the analysis of drugs and for analysis of behavior: we had identified a unique property of imipramine, and this property seemed to provide pharmacologic evidence that positive and negative reinforcement were in some respects different processes.

Fortunately, the research did not stop there. In our experiments with fixed-interval escape, shock had been delivered to the squirrel monkey through a floor grid. Under these conditions, the monkey could modify the effective shock level by changing its posture and thereby the portion of its body that came in contact with the grid. With the invaluable help of C.A. Gill, we had incorporated a variety of modifications in our procedures to circumvent this problem. The last of these was the construction of a new apparatus in which shock was delivered to the monkey through electrodes attached to its tail. In this apparatus, the monkey's behavior could not modify its contact with the shock source. When imipramine was administered under these conditions, the facilitative effect on responding that had been observed 24 hours after administration no longer occurred.

Other information was available to us. We knew that the rate of responding maintained by the fixed-interval schedule of escape increased with increases in shock level. At about the same time, Doctor Cook had independently begun studies of the effects of drugs on general activity, measured during fixed-interval positive reinforcement by the interruption of photocell beams at various locations within the experimental chamber. When imipramine was administered in that situation, it had relatively small effects on level of activity on the day of drug administration but produced increases relative to the baseline level 24 hours later (details are provided in Cook, 1965).

Now it was possible to interpret the various experimental outcomes. In the original apparatus, the shock had at least two effects: its termination maintained lever pressing, but the shock also elicited or maintained various activities or postures that modified the monkey's contact with the grid. In the final apparatus, the second of these effects was largely eliminated. In both conditions, imipramine also had at least two effects 24 hours after administration: it had a direct effect on responding maintained by negative reinforcement, presumably equivalent to its effect on responding maintained by positive reinforcement, and it produced an increase in the level of activity. In other words, the unique effect of imipramine was not a direct effect of this drug specifically on behavior maintained by negative reinforcement; instead, the administration of imipramine made it impossible, 24 hours later, for the monkey to sit still. Because the monkey could not maintain its postural adjustment to the grid, its changing contact with the grid was effectively equivalent to an increase in shock level and the rate of responding increased.

This experiment involved multiple functions of both the drug and the shock: the drug had an effect on reinforced responding and an eliciting effect on activity; the shock had an effect as a negative reinforcer and effects on posture that might be characterized as eliciting. Only by examining each of these effects and their interactions was it possible adequately to analyze the performance. And in the final analysis, it was at no time proper to treat the drug as anything other than a stimulus superimposed on performance.

To summarize, then: drugs are stimuli. They do have unique properties, but as we work with them we must hold before us a simple principle that nolds for all stimuli. The principle can be stated in two ways: stimuli have multiple functions—no stimulus has a single action.

REFERENCES

Catania, A.C. Reinforcement schedules and psychophysical judgments: A study of some temporal properties of behavior. In W.N. Schoenfeld, ed., *The Theory of Reinforcement Schedules*, New York, Appleton-Century-Crofts, 1970, 1-42.

Cook, L. Behavior changes with antipsychotic drugs in animals. In D. Bente and P.B. Bradley, eds., *Neuropsychopharmacology. Vol. 4.* Amsterdam, Elsevier, 1965, 91-99.

——and Catania, A.C. Effects of drugs on avoidance and escape behavior. *Fed. Proc.*, 1964, *23*, 818-835.

Discriminative Stimulus Functions of Drugs: Interpretations. II

J. Bruce Overmier

Department of Psychology
University of Minnesota
Minneapolis, Minnesota

Schuster and Brady (Chapter 8) have given us a very clear demonstration that both drugs *and* interoceptive stimulation in the form of infusion rate, per se, can function as discriminative stimuli for operants on a trial-to-trial basis. These drug observations then reinforce earlier suggestive reports by Cook et al. (1960). However, I find the infusion rate data most striking. Who could have guessed that increasing the fluid volume in the superior vena cava by something on the order of 1/10 of 1 percent could function as an adequate stimulus. Even Bykov would be impressed! This infusion data makes very clear that organisms are fantastically sensitive to variations in their internal milieu—certainly more so than to changes in their external environment if we refer to the available psychophysics data.

Harris and Balster (Chapter 7) have gone on to demonstrate again the greater sensitivity of the organism to its internal environment by showing that drugs at dosages of less than the standard pharmacologic ED_{50} can exert behavioral control. Their technique appears to be very sensitive—more so than Overton's T-maze technique (Chapter 6). This greater sensitivity is shown in two ways: (a) in general, Harris and Balster found smaller drug doses effective in behavior control, and (b) they found some behavioral transfer between atropine to its quaternary derivative. This latter difference might indicate, however, that Harris and Balster are looking at different phenomena than Overton, because Overton did not find evidence for such transfer. Stimulus control by drugs may well be very different than state-dependent learning though both have in common a dependence upon some drugs having different properties and effects. The former may be dependent upon peripheral effects while the latter may depend upon central effects.

Overton's T-maze technique with its emphasis upon first trial choice in each reversal has the most intuitive appeal to me. I suppose this is because I am a Tolmanian at heart. Overton's technique seems to be less sensitive than the other go-no-go and choice techniques reported. But this may have the advantage of enabling us to establish some gross classifications of drugs by their action in transfer tests of the type that have been reported here. Such transfer tests might occasionally have us group together some agents with widely differing pharmacologic properties. The transfer tests strike me as a particularly promising line of research. At the very least, they will reveal the dimensionality of the internal drug space.

Overton has attempted to eliminate peripheral proprioceptive changes as the mechanisms underlying his dissociation phenomenon. It is my guess that he has gone a long way toward achieving this goal—though the other two chapters make it clear that Ss can use such cues.

Perhaps the most striking feature of all the reported research is the potency of the drug operation in the control of behavior. In the tasks examined, the drug operations were clearly more powerful than most external stimulus operations tried. Furthermore, according to Harris and Balster's data, once discriminative control is established, it is difficult if not impossible to reverse. Such a phenomenon could have important implications for treatment of drug addiction, psychotherapy with tranquilized patients, and for such esoteric topics as learning theory.

Do the internal drug-induced variations have some sort of privileged status regarding behavior control when compared to external stimuli? There are precedents for hypothesizing that these drug-state stimuli might have such privileged status. For example, Garcia and Koelling (1966) have clearly shown that not all external discriminable stimuli are equally good cues for a given event; gustatory and olfactory stimuli are rapidly established as cues for internal discomfort but not for peripheral pain, while auditory and visual stimuli are easily established as cues for peripheral pain but not for internal malaise. Similarly, Dobrzecka, Szwejkowska, and Konorski (1966) have shown differential effectiveness of qualitative and directional cues with respect to the learning of go-no-go and choice tasks. In the former, stimulus quality dominated, while in the latter, stimulus orientation dominated. Konorski (1967) has suggested that this difference lies in the organization of the integrative mechanisms of the brain. Indeed, Herrick (1948) has described such integrative mechanisms in the medulla that could account for Garcia's findings.

Overton has mentioned here and other places two possible explanatory mechanisms for the observed phenomena. One is a simple stimulus mechanism and one appeals to organizational *changes* in the brain. While some effects of the induced drug states are functionally homologous with external stimulus phenomena and the cast of this book is to emphasize these, there are some data problems for the simple stimulus model. For example, the asymmetrical dissociation effects reported by Overton do not jibe with the notion of stimulus generalization. Similarly, the failure to find generalization decrements going from pentobarbital to phenobarbital to ethyl alcohol to meprobamate (Overton, 1966) can be considered a problem for the stimulus model.

On the other hand, if the learning set effect that Overton hinted at could be demonstrated to be a reliable phenomenon over a wide range of *pairs* of drugs to other *pairs* of drugs, and the pairs had previously failed to show transfer to each other, then the stimulus model would gain additional credence.

Let me suggest an experiment that might discriminate between a stimulus mechanism and an organizational mechanism with several independent states. In the typical choice experiment described today, under Drug A, $R_a \to S^R$ and under Drug B, $R_b \to S^R$, and the reinforcement was the same in both cases (see Fig. 1). Now consider the following variation. Under Drug A, $R_a \to S_a^R$ (say food) and under Drug B, $R_b \to S_a^R$ (say sucrose). Will learning of the problem be faster when there are unique reinforcers asso-

Experimental Operations	Stimulus Functions
Drug A → R_a → S_g^R Drug B → R_b → S_g^R	$S_a \to r_g - s_g \to R_a$ $S_b \to r_g - s_g \to R_b$
Drug A → R_a → S_a^R Drug B → R_b → S_b^R	$S_a \to r_a - s_a \to R_a$ $S_b \to r_b - s_b \to R_b$

Fig. 1. Symbolic representation of the standard drug-discrimination task and the assumed functional properties of the drug according to a simple stimulus model (top). This is to be contrasted with the similar analysis of the proposed discriminative choice task using unique reinforcers for each response chain. The symbols $r_g - s_g$, $r_a - s_a$, and $r_b - s_b$ refer to evoked anticipatory goal reactions and their associated feedback (expectancies).

ciated with the two drug states? If we are dealing with independent organizational mechanisms, the two versions should be learned equally fast. This is because drug controlled independent organizational mechanisms would prevent the common reinforcement expectancy ($r_g - s_g$) from evoking simultaneously both R_a and R_b. However, if the drugs are functioning as stimuli, then the unique reinforcer version should be learned faster. This is because in the second problem the two drugs elicit unique expectancies (and their feedback stimuli), whereas in the first problem, the two drugs elicit the same expectancy. Hence in the first task, generalization between the drug conditions is enhanced by the common expectancy resulting in slower acquisition. This phenomenon has been demonstrated for "real" stimuli (Trapold, 1970) and should also be true for drug-induced states if the stimulus model is correct.

Finally, it should be noted that Girden, who is generally recognized as giving us the first clear demonstration of "dissociation" under curare which is now called state-dependent learning (Girden and Culler, 1937), also has demonstrated that the dissociation phenomenon is dependent upon certain cortical areas being intact. Girden (1940) reported that certain restricted bilateral ablations eliminated the dissociation effect, and CRs freely transferred from drugged state to undrugged and *vice versa*. This can be taken to suggest direct surgical intrusion as a fruitful line of research in the study of the apparent stimulus control by drugs. It may even reveal the drugs' sites of psychoactivity.

REFERENCES

Cook, L., Davidson, D.J., and Kelleher, R.T. Epinephrine, norepinephrine, and acetylcholine as conditioned stimuli for avoidance behavior. *Science*, 1960, *131*, 990-991.

Dobrzecka, C., Szwejokowska, G., and Konorski, J. Qualitative versus directional cues in two forms of differentiation. *Science*, 1966, *153*, 87-89.

Garcia, J., and Koelling, R.A. Relation of cue to consequence in avoidance learning. *Psychonomic Science*, 1966, *4*, 123-124.

Girden, E. Cerebral mechanisms in conditioning under curare. *Amer. J. Psychol.*, 1940, *53*, 397-406.

—— and Culler, E. Conditioned responses in curarized striate muscle in dogs. *J. Comp. Psychol.*, 1937, *23*, 261-274.

Herrick, C.J. *The Brain of the Tiger Salamander, Ambystoma Tigrinum*. Chicago, University of Chicago Press, 1948.

Konorski, J. *The Integrative Activity of the Brain*. Chicago, University of Chicago Press, 1967.

Overton, D.A. State-dependent learning produced by depressant and atropine-like drugs. *Psychopharmacologia (Berl.)*, 1966, *10*, 6-31

Trapold, M.A. Are expectancies based upon different positive reinforcing events discriminably different? *Learning and Motivation*, 1970, *1*, 129-140.

SECTION 4

REINFORCING STIMULUS FUNCTIONS OF DRUGS

10

Opiates as Reinforcing Stimuli[1]

James H. Woods* and Charles R. Schuster**

*Department of Pharmacology
 University of Michigan
 Ann Arbor, Michigan
**Department of Psychiatry
 University of Chicago
 Chicago, Illinois

Morphine is the principle derivative of opium and the prototypic opiate for a great deal of pharmacologic investigation. One way to examine the significance of the behavioral properties of morphine and other opiates is to investigate the manner in which they modify and strengthen behavior. If intravenous morphine or other opiates are presented immediately following a response and the response frequency increases, then opiates can be said to serve as reinforcers. This proposition supposes that morphine and morphine-like drugs might act as reinforcers in the absence of setting conditions (e.g., drug deprivation and conditioning history). Other reinforcers (e.g., intracranial stimulation and changes in illumination) appear to have such properties.

The proposition that opiates can act as reinforcers without previous conditioning history or drug deprivation conditions brings with it a number of methodological and empirical difficulties. The reinforcement process is measured by behavioral change occurring through time. However, morphine's behavioral effects also change over time, that is, tolerance develops to successive doses. For example, response output maintained by food presentation is decreased by morphine administration and with successive administrations there is a diminution of this behavioral effect (e.g., McMillan and Morse, 1967). Some investigators have assumed that tolerance also

[1] The research reported here was supported by NIMH Grant 5-R10-12084 to the University of Michigan, M.H. Seevers, principle investigator.

develops to the reinforcing property of barbiturates (Davis and Miller, 1963) though this hypothesis requires more direct empirical support.

Physical dependence and reinforcing efficacy of opiates. A more serious difficulty in testing our proposition arises with the development of physical dependence to morphine on chronic administration. Physical dependence on morphine and morphine-like drugs is demonstrated when chronic drug administration is abruptly terminated and vast patterns of behavioral, somatic, sympathetic, and parasympathetic changes, termed the withdrawal syndrome, ensue. A discussion of the properties and parameters of physical dependence and the withdrawal syndrome is beyond the scope of this presentation. However, for the rhesus monkey, the subjects used in the experiments described here, physical dependence and the withdrawal syndrome have been described in detail elsewhere (Seevers and Deneau, 1963). Subsequent morphine administration can reduce the signs of the morphine withdrawal syndrome. Since morphine sustains physical dependence and reduces the opiate withdrawal syndrome, some investigators have argued that morphine may derive its reinforcing efficacy from its ability to reduce or postpone the hypothesized withdrawal-induced stimulation (e.g., Nichols, 1965; Weeks, 1962). While the withdrawal syndrome has been described by human addicts as subjectively similar to an intense case of influenza, there is as yet no direct evidence that morphine-dependent animals self-administer morphine to terminate such hypothesized stimulation.

Thus, behavioral and other general counteradaptations to repeated administration of morphine may interact with the measurement of morphine's reinforcing efficacy. If physical dependence were necessary for morphine to act as a positive reinforcer, it should be impossible to maintain an operant response with morphine presentations in the absence of physical dependence. If, on the other hand, morphine is a reinforcer in the absence of physical dependence, morphine may function as a reinforcer in a more general manner. There are two experimental implications of this suggestion. Assessment of the role of physical dependence in determining the reinforcing strength of morphine is facilitated. Further, in the absence of physical dependence, the use of morphine as a reinforcer can provide a relatively simple preparation for investigating other variables influencing its reinforcing strength.

The extent to which physical dependence is separable from the reinforcing property of morphine is a prime consideration. Previous investigations have usually omitted the necessary observations for evaluating this possibility by giving noncontingent morphine injections to insure physical dependence prior to a test of morphine's reinforcing efficacy (Nichols, 1965; Thompson and Schuster, 1964; Weeks, 1962). There is little doubt that subsequent to physical dependence development, morphine will maintain operant responding. For example, Thompson and Schuster (1964) found that morphine-dependent rhesus monkeys maintained responding on a chained reinforcement schedule in which morphine infusion was the terminal stimulus event. Although low overall response rates were observed, patterns of responding in the fixed-interval and fixed-ratio components of the chained schedule resembled patterns maintained by other reinforcers (Ferster and Skinner, 1957).

Morphine self-administration without prior drug treatment. In the first of the experiments (Schuster, 1970), initial noncontingent morphine administration was eliminated and rhesus monkeys, following internal jugular catheterization[2], were exposed to response-contingent morphine presentations. Response-contingent saline injections of equal volume (0.2 ml/kg) served as the five-day control baseline. Figure 1 shows, for three rhesus monkeys, the rate of bar pressing when a 1.0 mg/kg injection of morphine sulfate was delivered following each lever press over the course of a 30-day exposure to morphine. When saline presentations were response contingent, a mean of five responses per 24-hour period were emitted. Response rates for morphine presentations increased to 30 to 45 per 24-hour period by the end of the 30-day period.

There is little question that morphine was serving as a reinforcer at the end of this period. There are, however, several peculiarities of these data. The response rates were very low. Since response rates increased very slowly over the 30-day period and rose above saline control rates only after six to eight days, morphine cannot be confirmed as a reinforcer until that time. While this experiment shows that prior noncontingent morphine administration is not necessary to demonstrate reinforcing capabilities of morphine, it was unclear whether the reinforcement criterion was met *prior* to the development of physical dependence on morphine.

Self-administration of low morphine doses. Morphine physical dependence is dose-related, and the optimal procedure for its development is to administer doses to maintain blood levels continuously. However, the subcutaneous administration of 3 mg/kg every six hours is sufficient to develop near maximum dependence in the rhesus monkey (Seevers and Deaneau, 1963). Using this drug regimen, dependence grows to a maximum at around 30 days, as evidenced by the withdrawal syndrome on abrupt cessation of morphine administration. It is also possible to elicit a weaker form of withdrawal after only 14 days following initiation of the drug regimen. In relation to the data presented in Figure 1, it is not clear whether a rein-

---

[2] Details of the catheterization procedure and catheter-protection devices are available from the authors.

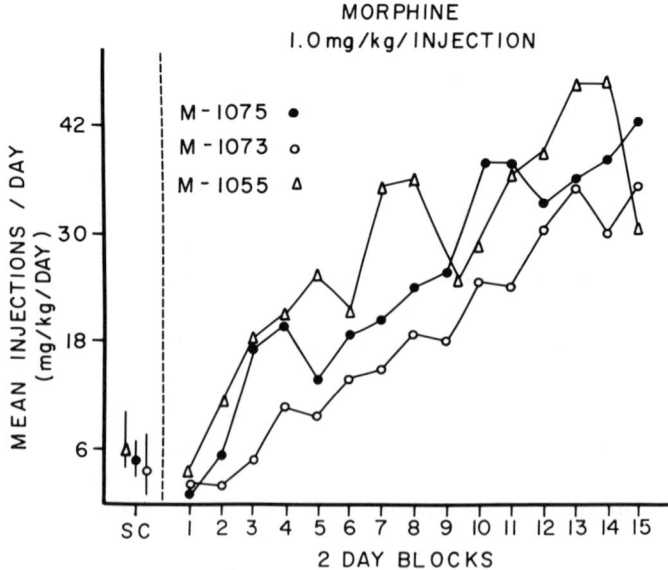

Fig. 1. The number of injections per 24-hour period over a 30-day exposure to 1 mg/kg/injection of morphine sulfate. The individual response frequency of the monkeys are represented by the parameters.

forcing effect occurred prior to significant development of physical dependence. When large doses of morphine are used as reinforcers, the reinforcement process and the development of physical dependence may coincide.

On the other hand, when very small doses of morphine (100 µg/kg) are given subcutaneously every six hours, morphine dependence cannot be detected by observational techniques when the dose regimen is abruptly terminated (Seevers and Deneau, 1963). Thus, if a very small dose of morphine is used, it might be possible to maintain responding for morphine presentations prior to and, perhaps, in the absence of physical dependence. Since a detailed report of investigations on this and related work has been presented elsewhere (Schuster, 1968; Woods and Schuster, 1968), only a relevant portion will be emphasized here. Five monkeys prepared with intravenous catheters were conditioned to respond on a 2.5-minute variable-interval schedule of food reinforcement for intravenous morphine presentations. The availability of drug or food was indicated by the illumination of lights mounted directly in front of the monkey. Morphine presentations were made available during each of four equally spaced one-hour periods. One-hour periods of food availability bounded each period of morphine availability. Water was available at all times on a continuous reinforcement

Table 1. *Responses per minute under the various conditions of the experiment for the five monkeys* [*]

Monkeys	M6		M7		M841		M1086		M2031	
mcg/kg/inj.	10	1,000	10	1,000	25	1,000	10	250	10	1,000
S.C.	0.10	0.15	0.11	0.18	0.00	0.07	0.11	0.24	0.01	0.09
Conditions D 1-3	0.80	0.04	0.29	0.03	1.60	0.22	0.31	0.24	1.19	0.07
D 4-6	0.40	0.02	0.45	0.03	1.53	0.16	0.27	0.24	2.80	0.09
D 7-9	0.80	0.04	0.34	0.04	1.12	0.21	0.41	0.18	3.24	0.22
D 10-12	0.53	0.04	0.43	0.05	1.67	0.32	0.75	0.32	1.94	0.39
D 13-15	0.54	0.12	0.45	0.07	1.30	0.36	0.34	0.35	1.95	0.46
Ext. 1-3	0.33	2.60	0.20	9.62	0.14	0.89	0.13	1.41	1.19	0.48
Ext. 4-6	0.23	1.75	0.14	2.41	0.05	0.10	0.15	0.53	0.54	0.26

[*] D 1-15 represent the mean drug-lever responses per minute averaged in three-day intervals for the fifteen-day test periods at the lowest and highest dosage levels of morphine. Ext. 1-3 and Ext. 4-6 represent the mean drug-lever responses per minute for the two successive three-day periods following each dosage level of morphine in which saline was substituted. S.C.=Average responses per minute for saline presentations for the five days prior to exposure to morphine. Monkeys M6 and M7 were exposed to the high dose initially; M841, M1086, and M2031 were exposed to the low dose initially.

schedule. Each dose/injection (10, 25, 100, 250, 500, 1,000 µg/kg/injection) was tested for 15 days, with saline replacing morphine for at least 10 days before another dose was tested. Table 1 shows the mean response rates for each monkey at the highest and lowest doses tested. There were small but reliable increases in response rate with the lowest dose for each of the five monkeys within the first three days of exposure. The response rate increases for low doses of morphine presentation were maintained throughout the 15-day exposure to this dose. When saline presentations were substituted, response rates decreased and, in most cases, approximated the response rate prior to morphine exposure. The reduction in behavior maintained by food and water presentations due to morphine is displayed in Table 2 for one of the monkeys. The low dose of morphine had little if any effect on these behaviors during the 15-day exposure period or when morphine presentations were discontinued.

The four monkeys exposed to 10 µg/kg/injection received on the average 310 µg/kg/day, and, it will be recalled, a dose of over 400 µg/kg/day is necessary to produce recognizable indications of withdrawal within this period (Seevers and Deneau, 1963). Therefore when low doses/injection of morphine are used, it is possible to observe reinforcement effects at doses/day below those necessary to produce physical dependence.

Quite different effects were obtained when the monkeys were exposed to high unit doses. Response rates leading to morphine presentation were initially either unchanged or slightly depressed. The rates of responding increased above saline control level over the 15-day exposure to this high unit-dose for three of the five monkeys so that at the end of this period rates

Table 2. *Response output ratios for food presentations on a variable-interval schedule and water reinforcement on a continuous reinforcement schedule.* *

Sequence of Conditions	Food		Water	
	10 µg/kg	1000 µg/kg	10 µg/kg	1000 µg/kg
Saline	0.85-1.11	0.82-1.08	0.88-1.06	0.93-1.14
D 1-3	0.76	1.07	1.02	0.85
D 4-6	0.89	0.00	0.80	0.69
D 7-9	0.65	0.18	0.80	0.72
D 10-12	0.84	0.28	0.95	0.71
D 13-15	0.81	0.30	0.95	0.82
Saline 1	0.81	0.00	0.98	0.58
Saline 2	0.85	0.14	1.04	1.48
Saline 3	0.71	0.22	0.82	2.65
Saline 4	0.91	0.89	0.82	1.40
Saline 5	0.96	1.60	0.87	1.21

*The ratios are computed by taking the five-day average rate of responding prior to the introduction of morphine as a unity. The daily range of variation under saline conditions prior to the introduction of morphine is indicated by the initial entry, labeled Saline. D 1-3 through D 13-15 indicate the average three-day output ratios under conditions of self-administration of morphine (10 or 1,000 µg/kg/inj). The last entries in the table are daily averaged output ratios for the first five days under saline self-administration subsequent to exposure to morphine. Data presented are those of M2031 (Table 1).

of responding were higher than those based upon saline presentations. Note that these three monkeys were exposed to lower doses initially. The diminished effect of the high doses with these monkeys has been due to the development of tolerance to the rate of decreasing effects of morphine.

The low response rates for the 1 mg/kg unit-dose of morphine are consistent with those presented in Figure 1. Response output for food and water presentations was also depressed by response-contingent morphine (Table 2). There was likewise a return of these behaviors toward saline control conditions. These trends toward increases in responding based on morphine, food, and water presentations appear related to the development of tolerance to the rate-decreasing properties of the drug. When morphine was discontinued (i.e., extinction was initiated), there was a transitory decreased rate of responding maintained by food and water presentations. Both these trends indicate the development of physical dependence and were correlated with withdrawal signs. Other observations of operant responding during withdrawal from morphine are consistent with these data (Thompson and Schuster, 1964; Schuster and Woods, 1968). The transitory increases in morphine responding during initial extinction following high morphine doses may have been a joint function of the development of physical dependence, the elimination of the depressant effects of morphine, and possible differences in reinforcing potency related to dose. Following exposure to low doses, where physical dependence and the depressant properties of morphine were eliminated, increases in extinction responding were not observed. If responding during initial extinction is used as a criterion of reinforcing efficacy, increases in reinforcing potency are conferred by increasing unit doses. Reinforcing effects at high doses are likely to be overridden by the rate-decreasing effects of morphine when response rate for morphine presentation is used as the criterion of reinforcement potency.

Rate reducing effects of opiates. Rates of responding maintained by the lower doses of morphine were, in all cases, quite modest and never approximated the response rates maintained by food presentation on the equal-valued variable-interval schedule (Table 1). It may be inevitable that when morphine is used as a reinforcer, dose-related behavioral effects interact with morphine's reinforcing efficacy in an opposing fashion. One tactic leading to a greater separation of these proposed behavioral effects is the use of schedules more resistant to morphine's rate-decreasing properties.

That schedule-engendered response rates are differentially decreased by morphine has been shown by McMillan and Morse (1967) in the pigeon. High rates of responding, maintained by fixed-ratio response requirements for food presentation, were suppressed less than the lower rates of responding, maintained by a fixed-interval reinforcement schedule. Low rates of food-reinforced responding are also more susceptible to morphine-induced rate decrements than are high rates of responding in rhesus monkeys (Woods, 1969). To generate differences in response rate, a multiple reinforcement schedule (Ferster and Skinner, 1957) was used with a fixed-interval component of eight minutes and a fixed-ratio schedule of 50 responses. One-minute time-out periods separated the components. Mean control response rates were 1.3 responses/sec in the fixed-interval component and 4.0 responses/sec in the fixed-ratio component. Figure 2 indicates that through a considerable dose range, fixed-interval low-rate responding was relatively more depressed than the higher rates engendered by the fixed-ratio schedule. Doses of morphine were administered subcutaneously once weekly. With this dose regimen, dose effects could be replicated, reducing the possibility that morphine tolerance played a role in the dose-response relation.

Methadone and codeine, two narcotic agents differing considerably from morphine in their general depressant and physical dependence-producing potential in the rhesus monkey (Seevers and Deneau, 1963) were chosen to compare to morphine's rate-decreasing effects. The rate-decreasing effects of these three narcotics are shown in Figure 3. As can be seen, in the suppression of fixed-ratio responding, morphine and methadone were similar in potency and codeine was far less potent than either methadone or morphine. There is some species generality to these rate-decreasing effects since the ranks of these agents are in the same order for the pigeon (Woods, 1969).

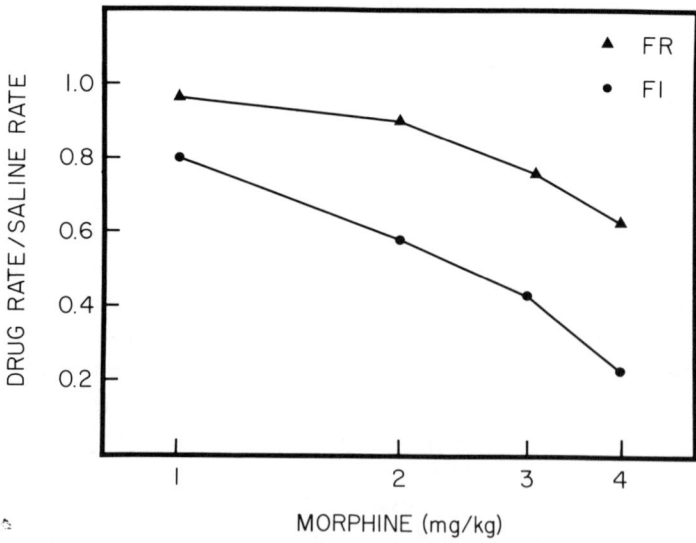

Fig. 2. Response-output ratio as related to subcutaneous administration of morphine sulfate in the fixed-interval (FI) and fixed-ratio (FR) components of a multiple schedule of reinforcement. Two observations were obtained at each dose in each of two monkeys. The drug-saline ratios were averaged for the purpose of computing the data points.

Perhaps the rate-decreasing properties of these drugs are predictive of the relative rates of responding when these agents are used as reinforcers. At

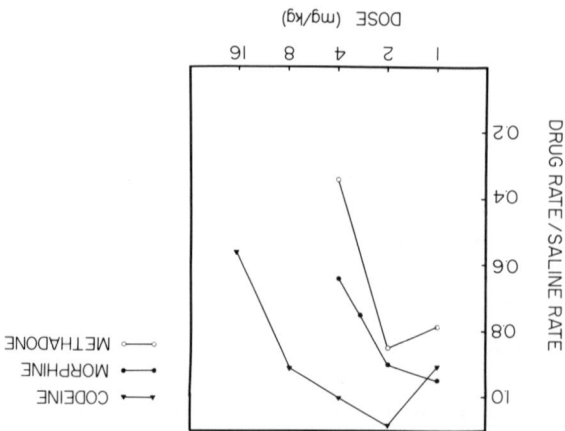

Fig. 3. Response output as related to subcutaneous administration of morphine sulfate, codeine phosphate, and methadone hydrochloride in the fixed-ratio component of a multiple fixed-interval and fixed-ratio schedule of reinforcement. Two observations were obtained at each dose in each of two monkeys. The dose-saline ratios were averaged for observation.

equivalent doses/injection, morphine and methadone should generate closely equivalent but lower rates of self-administration than codeine if this is the case. Fixed-ratio responding for drug was used to test this notion. Cocaine was used to engender baseline performance since it readily generates schedule-controlled patterns of responding (Pickens and Thompson, 1968) and since it affords comparison to another class of pharmacologic agents, viz., psychomotor stimulants. There is little or no cross-tolerance between cocaine and opiates (Seevers and Deneau, 1963) and cocaine does not influence the development of morphine physical dependence (McCarthy, 1960).

A session was initiated by the illumination of a white house-light and terminated following the 35th reinforcement or when four hours elapsed, whichever occurred first. With each injection, the white light extinguished, a green light signalled drug infusion, followed by a one-minute time-out. The ratio-requirement for each drug infusion was raised to and maintained at 20

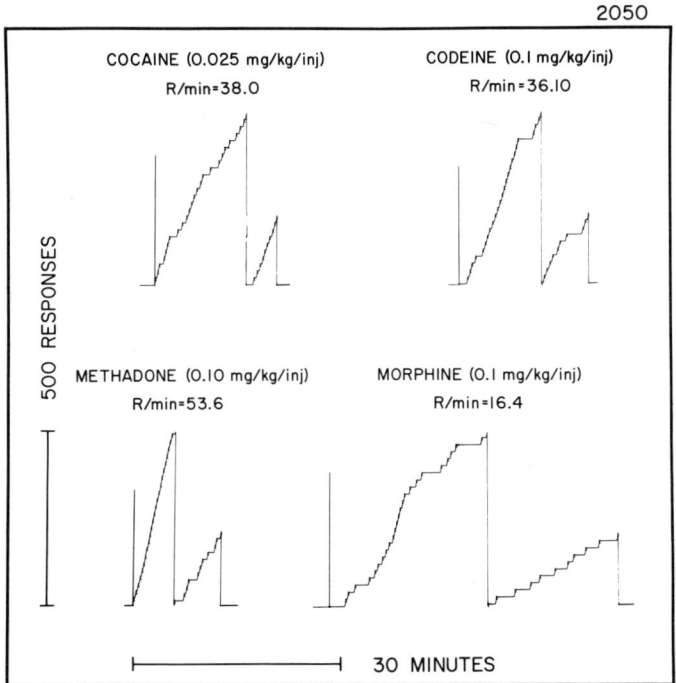

Fig. 4. Fixed-ratio responding for cocaine hydrochloride, morphine sulfate, codeine phosphate, methadone hydrochloride presented intravenously. Individual responses step the recording pen upward. The deflection of the pen indicates delivery of drug. The recorder did not advance in time during the infusion of drug or during the time-out period.

responses/injection. When behavior stabilized, saline was substituted for cocaine and responding in extinction observed. Then morphine, methadone, and codeine were substituted for saline. Each drug was available for five sessions followed by saline substitution usually for two to three sessions. Figure 4 presents cumulative records for one monkey on the terminal day of self-administration of the four agents. Codeine and cocaine generate nearly equivalent self-administration rates while morphine is self-administered at much lower rates and methadone sustains the highest rate. Patterns of responding were much like those one might expect with fixed-ratio responding for food presentation or for the termination of stimuli associated with shock, although overall response rates are slightly lower.

Data have been presented suggesting that the rate-increasing and maintaining effects of codeine, methadone, and morphine in self-administration are not related directly to their rate-decreasing effects on behavior maintained by food presentations. Before drawing a firm conclusion on this point, it will be necessary to use equivalent reinforcement schedules generating comparable rates of responding in the same organism.

Kolb and DuMez (1931) demonstrated that single daily injections of codeine for periods of up to one year at doses up to 30 times that administered in these experiments do not produce dependence in the monkey. Seevers (1936) found that codeine given to rhesus monkeys in single daily injections at 10 times the total daily dose used in this experiment, produced no withdrawal syndrome when the drug was discontinued after 21 months of administration. Likewise, methadone administered once each day for 96 days (Woods, Wyngaarden, and Seevers, 1947) and three times each day for 142 days (Cochin, Gruhzit, Woods, and Seevers, 1948) at two to three times the total daily dose given in this situation produced no recognizable indications of withdrawal symptoms when the drug regimen was abruptly stopped. These data lend considerable credence to the argument that morphine and morphine-like drugs can act as reinforcers at dosages below those necessary to produce physical dependence.

Higher overall response rates were observed in the present experiment for morphine presentations than in the previously reported experiments. Probably, both the use of a fixed-ratio schedule and a single brief exposure to the drug each day contributed to the higher overall response rates observed in this experiment, suggesting that it is necessary to use widely spaced sessions with small drug doses if physical dependence is to be obviated.

Effect of naloxone on cocaine and codeine self-administration. Schedule-controlled response rates and patterns can be a prime determinant of the behavioral effects of drugs (Kelleher and Morse, 1968). It has been argued that with some drugs, response rates are a more important controlling variable than the type of event (e.g., food presentation or electric shock termination) that maintains responding (Kelleher and Morse, 1964). Since rates and patterns of responding maintained by codeine and cocaine were very similar (Fig. 4), it was appropriate to compare the effects of another drug on responding reinforced by agents from different pharmacologic classes. The effects of naloxone were assessed. Naloxone is a narcotic antagonist that counteracts many of the effects of opiates (Martin, 1967), and naloxone as well diminishes the rate-decreasing effects of morphine (McMillan, 1969; Woods, 1969). As can be seen in Figure 5, naloxone administration had no effect on cocaine-reinforced responding. Following naloxone administration when codeine was the reinforcer, responding ceased after three injections for that session. One possible effect of naloxone may have been to antagonize the reinforcing property of codeine, thus effectively creating extinction conditions. Extinction sessions (i.e., when saline is substituted for drug) usually yield a greater response output than that observed. In addition, an interesting possibility is that the administration of naloxone created conditions in which codeine was aversive. In subsequent experiments, unpublished observations on codeine-naloxone interactions have borne out the reliability of the above findings, and other narcotic drugs have shown

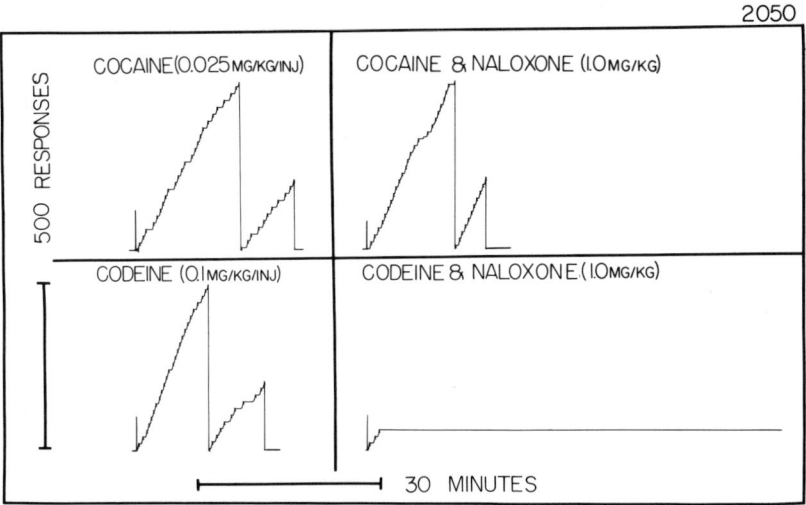

Fig. 5. The effects of naloxone administration on responding maintained by cocaine and codeine presentations. Naloxone was administered intravenously immediately prior to the beginning of the session. Individual responses step the recording pen upward. The deflection of the pen indicates delivery of drug. The recorder did not advance in time during the infusion of drug or during the time-out period.

similar interactions with naloxone. Furthermore, nalorphine, another opiate antagonist, produces changes in morphine-reinforced responding (Goldberg, Woods, and Schuster, 1968). Thus, at least some narcotic antagonists effect changes in behavior that depend upon the kind of drug used as a reinforcer. Whether other drugs will also interact with drug reinforcers in specific manners is both an interesting and open question.

The primary proposition of this chapter has been that morphine and morphine-like drugs can function as reinforcers without previous conditioning history or drug deprivation conditions. Experimental evidence was presented indicating that some opiates (e.g., codeine and methadone) with weak potential for producing physical dependence in single daily injections are stronger reinforcers by rate-maintenance measures than morphine. Even morphine, which has strong physical dependence producing potential, is a weak reinforcer at doses below those necessary to produce dependence. Thus, it appears that the reinforcing property of the opiates may be more general than their physical dependence producing property. If this is the case, the role of physical dependence in modulating rates of self-administration is by no means clear. One of the reasons for this uncertainty is that as larger drug doses are administered and, hence, greater physical dependence is produced, there is concomitant general reduction of response output. Providing the drug during only a small portion of each day and using schedules that engenders high rates, tend to increase response strength. Another method of separating the reinforcing and rate-decreasing effects of these drugs is to use chained reinforcement schedules (Ferster and Skinner, 1957) in which the initial components are maintained by stimuli associated with drug infusion and the terminal member is drug infusion. The two studies (Thompson and Schuster, 1964; Schuster and Woods, 1968) that have investigated stimuli associated with drug infusion have shown powerful effects of such stimuli. Until the rate-decreasing effects of drug infusion are experimentally separated from their reinforcing or rate-maintaining effects, the question of the role of physical dependence will be to some extent mixed with the depressant properties of the drug. Tests of physical dependence produced by termination of response-contingent drug infusion are by definition confounded with extinction phenomena. Thus, it would be useful to employ behaviors maintained by a drug and, as well, by another reinforcer. If these behaviors are maintained in equal strength, so that the reinforcers maintain equivalent rates and patterns of responding, considerable refinement may be given to the analysis of physical dependence as a potential source of an opiate's reinforcing efficacy.

REFERENCES

Cochin, J., Gruhzit, C.C., Woods, L.A., and Seevers, M.H. Further observations on addiction to methadone in the monkey. *Proc. Soc. Exp. Biol. Med.*, 1948, *69*, 430.
Davis, J.D., and Miller, N.E. Fear and pain: Their effect on self-injection of amobarbital sodium in rats. *Science*, 1963, *141*, 1286.
Ferster, C.B., and Skinner, B.F. *Schedules of Reinforcement.* New York, Appleton-Century-Crofts, 1957.
Goldberg, S.R., Woods, J.H. and Schuster, C.R. Nalorphine-induced changes in morphine self-administration in rhesus monkeys. *Fed. Proc.*, 1968, *27*, 754.
Kelleher, R.T., and Morse, W.H. Escape behavior and punished behavior. *Fed. Proc.*, 1964, *23*, 808.
────── and Morse, W.H. Determinants of the specificity of behavioral effects of drugs. *Ergebn. Physiol.*, 1968, *60*, 1.
Kolb, L., and DuMez, A.G. Experimental addiction of animals to opiates. *U.S. Public Health Reports*, 1931, *46*, 698.
Martin, W.R. Opioid antagonists. *Pharmacol. Rev.*, 1967, *19*, 463.
McCarthy, D.A. Pharmacologic analysis of mechanism in morphine dependent state. *Dissertation Abstracts*, 1960, *20*, 4683.
McMillan, D.E. Behavioral interactions of naloxone with morphine and cyclozocine in the pigeon. *Fed. Proc.*, 1969, *28*, 736.
────── and Morse, W.H. Some effects of morphine and morphine antagonists on schedule-controlled behavior. *J. Pharmacol. Exp. Ther.*, 1967, *157*, 175.
Nichols, J.R. How opiates change behavior. *Sci. Amer.*, 1965, *212*, 80.
Pickens, R., and Thompson, T. Cocaine-reinforced behavior in rats: Effects of reinforcement magnitude and fixed ratio size. *J. Pharmacol. Exp. Ther.*, 1968, *161*, 122.
Schuster, C.R. Psychological approaches to opiate dependence and self-administration by laboratory animals. *Fed. Proc.*, 1970, *29*, 2-5.
────── Variables affecting the self-administration of drugs by rhesus monkeys. In Vagtborg, H., ed., *Use of Nonhuman Primates in Drug Evaluation.* Austin, University of Texas Press, 1968, 283.
────── and Woods, J.H. The conditioned reinforcing effects of stimuli associated with morphine reinforcement. *International Journal of the Addictions*, 1968, *3*, 223.
Seevers, M.H. Opiate addictions in the monkey. II. Dilaudid in comparison to morphine, heroin, and codeine. *J. Pharmacol. Exp. Ther.*, 1936, *56*, 157.
────── and Deneau, G.A. Physiological aspects of tolerance and physical dependence. In W.S. Rott and F.G. Hoffman, eds., *Physiological Pharmacology*, New York, Academic Press, Inc., 1963, *1*, 565.
Thompson, T., and Schuster, C.R. Morphine self-administration, food-reinforced and avoidance behaviors in rhesus monkeys. *Psychopharmacologia*, 1964, *5*, 87.
Weeks, J.R. Experimental morphine addiction: Method for automatic intravenous injections in unrestrained rats. *Science*, 1962, *138*, 143.
Woods, J.H. Effects of morphine, methadone and codeine on schedule-controlled behavior in the pigeon and rhesus monkey. *Fed. Proc.*, 1969, *28*, 511.
────── and Schuster, C.R. Reinforcement properties of morphine, cocaine, and SPA as a function of unit dose. *International Journal of the Addictions*, 1968, *3*, 231.
Woods, L.A., Wyngaarden, J.B., and Seevers, M.H. Addiction potentialities of 1, 1-diphenyl-1-(b-dimethylaminopropyl)-butanone-2 hydrochloride (amidone) in the monkey. *Proc. Soc. Exp. Biol. Med.*, 1947, *65*, 113.

Characteristics of Stimulant Drug Reinforcement[1]

Roy Pickens and Travis Thompson

Departments of Psychiatry and Pharmacology
University of Minnesota
Minneapolis, Minnesota

A number of stimuli serve as reinforcers for operant behavior. These stimuli unify the many and varied responses leading to their presentation, and make the behavioral unit formed more likely to recur. Apart from these effects, however, reinforcers seemingly have little else in common. They differ physically over a wide range, including such dissimilar events as food, light and novel stimulus presentation, electric shock termination, and electrical stimulation of the brain. It is not surprising therefore that the functional properties of reinforcers also differ. In fact, each reinforcer appears to have a set of unique characteristics. In the present chapter, some of the characteristics of stimulant drugs as reinforcers are examined, with special consideration given to the behavior of the organism under such conditions and to factors influencing this behavior.

STIMULANT DRUGS

Stimulant drugs directly stimulate the central nervous system, producing increased excitability and motor activity, decreased food intake and fatigue, and, for humans at least, elevation of mood (Goth, 1968; Kosman and Unna, 1968). These effects do not occur equally for all of the drugs, however, and chronic administration or overdosage may produce different effects (Weiss and Laties, 1962). Many stimulants also possess sympathomimetic activity,

---

[1] Preparation of this chapter was supported in part by USPHS Research Grants No. MH-14112 and MH-15349 to the University of Minnesota.

producing increased blood pressure and heart rate, dilation of the pupils, and so forth (Ellis, 1956). In sharp contrast to opiate and barbiturate drugs, stimulants do not produce physical dependence, and therefore no severe withdrawal symptoms following discontinuing drug administration. Tolerance to the stimulants is marked in some cases (e.g., amphetamines), but not evident in others, (e.g., cocaine) (Seevers and Deneau, 1963). The drugs apparently produce their similar effects through different biochemical mechanisms (Axelrod, 1959; Muscholl, 1966).

STIMULANTS AS REINFORCERS

A number of stimulants serve as reinforcers for operant behavior (Pickens, 1968). These drugs include, for the rat, d-amphetamine (Pickens and Thompson, 1967; Pickens and Harris, 1968), methamphetamine (Pickens, Meisch, and McGuire, 1967; McGuire, 1966; Pickens, Meisch, and Dougherty, 1968a), and cocaine (Pickens and Thompson, 1967; Pickens and Thompson, 1968), and, for the monkey, d-amphetamine and methamphetamine (Deneau, Yanagita, and Seevers, 1964), cocaine (Deaneau, Yanagita, and Seevers, 1964; Woods and Schuster, 1968), caffeine (Schuster, Woods, and Seevers, 1968), nicotine (Deaneau and Inoki, 1967; Jarvik, 1967), SPA[2] (Estrada, Villarreal, and Schuster, 1967; Woods and Schuster, 1968), fencamfamine[3] (Estrada, Villarreal, and Schuster, 1967), and methylphenidate, pipradrol, and phenmetrazine (Wilson, Hitomi, and Schuster, 1969). Recently pipradrol, methylphenidate, and tranylcypromine have also been found to be reinforcers for rats (Pickens, Plunkett, Jenkins, and Cherek, unpublished). The reinforcing doses of these drugs are summarized in Table 1.

The only stimulant drug tested which has not served as a reinforcer is

TABLE 1. *Reinforcing doses of stimulant drugs for animals*

Drug	Dose/Injection (in mg/kg)	
	Rat	Monkey
d-Amphetamine	0.25-1.0	0.25-0.1
Caffeine		1.0-5.0
Cocaine	0.25-3.0	0.05-1.2
Fencamfamin		0.1-2.0
Methamphetamine	0.25-2.0	0.1
Methylphenidate	0.25-0.5	0.05-0.4
Nicotine		0.025-2.0
Phenmetrazine		0.05-0.8
Pipradrol	1.5-3.0	0.05-0.4
SPA		0.05-1.0
Tranylcypromine	0.1-0.2	

[2] (1)-1-2-diphenyl1-1-dimethyl-aminoethane
[3] 2-phenyl-3-ethylaminobicylo-2,2,1-heptane

pemoline (Wilson, Hitomi, and Schuster, 1969). Apparently, while most of these drugs are reinforcers for animals, not all are under the conditions studied. It is interesting that the same stimulants which are reinforcers for rats and monkeys are also thought to be reinforcers for humans as well, since these drugs are all said to possess high "abuse liability" (Eddy, Halbach, Isbell, and Seevers, 1965).

DRUG SELF-ADMINISTRATION METHODOLOGY

The reinforcing effects of stimulants have been determined using drug self-administration techniques (Thompson and Pickens, 1968, 1970). With these techniques, animals are given the opportunity to inhale, drink, or inject themselves with a drug preparation. If a drug is self-administered at rates above operant level and/or is subject to reinforcement schedule control, it is said to be serving as a reinforcer, since it is maintaining the behavior leading to its administration. In all except one of the stimulant reinforcement studies, intravenous drug self-administration has been the method used. In these studies, animals are equipped with chronic jugular catheters which connect by protective tubing to remote drug infusion pumps (Davis, 1966; Yanagita, Deneau, and Seevers, 1965). By operating a switch in the cage, the animal can activate the pump and thereby receive (self-administer) a predetermined amount of drug solution injected directly into the bloodstream (see Fig. 1). In the only other study in this area (Jarvik, 1967), drug self-administration by inhalation was used. This technique is similar to that for intravenous injection, except that a response (sucking on an air tube)

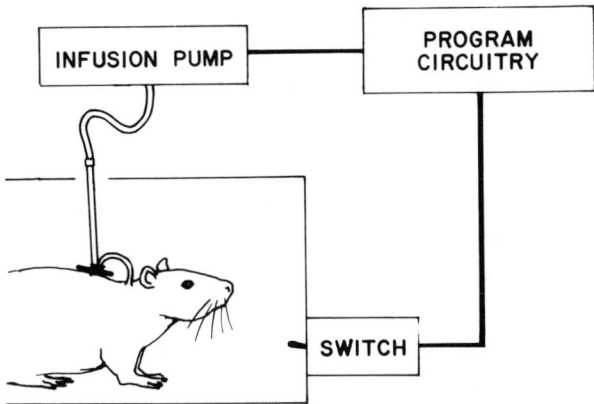

Fig. 1. Intravenous drug self-administration device for the rat.

ults in the drug being drawn into the lungs in the form of an air pension.

STIMULANT SELF-ADMINISTRATION BY RATS

The characteristics of stimulant drug reinforcement differ somewhat from those of other reinforcers. Some of the most detailed description of this behavior has come from studies of intravenous drug self-administration by rats (Pickens, 1968; Pickens, Meisch, and Dougherty, 1968a). In these studies, involving d-amphetamine, methamphetamine, and cocaine reinforcement, the drug is made available immediately after catheterization. Drug injections are programmed on a 24-hour continuous reinforcement schedule. A small cage light is illuminated during each injection to facilitate conditioning (which also occurs in the absence of the light, but more slowly). For the first several days, responding is infrequent and irregularly spaced. By the third or fourth day, the interval between successive self-administrations becomes more regular, perhaps with little change in hourly response rate. At this time evidence of conditioning is found, since drug removal produces extinction-like responding and intermittent reinforcement schedules can be maintained. The regularly spaced responding for drug injection ("patterning") produces an almost constant mg/kg/hour drug intake. The length of the interresponse interval is dose dependent, with higher drug doses producing longer intervals, and also drug dependent, with drugs with long durations of action (e.g., d-amphetamine) producing longer interresponse intervals than drugs with short duration of action (e.g., cocaine). Whereas before acquisition occurs occasional manual drug injections are given to prevent blood clotting in the catheter, forced drug injections do not noticeably facilitate conditioning. In fact, forced injections may delay conditioning, suggesting that such injections may be aversive to the animal.

BEHAVIORAL CHARACTERISTICS OF STIMULANT REINFORCEMENT

Following acquisition of drug self-administration behavior, alternating periods of drug intake and abstinence develop. During the drug-intake periods, response rate is low, with regularly spaced interresponse intervals, as shown in Figure 2. Such periods continue for 6 to 48 hours, varying to some

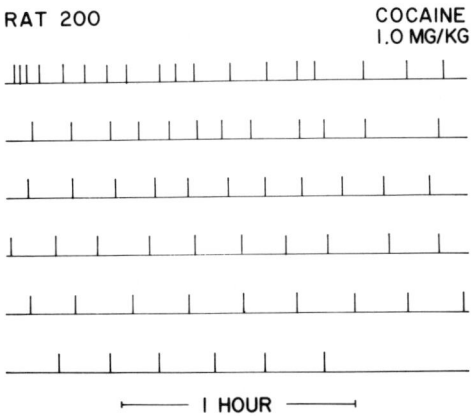

Fig. 2. Events record of responding during 11.3-hour drug-intake period for 1.0 mg/kg cocaine reinforcement. Each pip indicates a self-administration response.

extent with the drug used. Longer drug-intake periods are seen with drugs having long duration of action (e.g., d-amphetamine). Termination of a drug-intake period occurs abruptly, without evidence of satiation or extinction effects. A drug abstinence period follows, continuing for 2 to 24 hours. The length of the abstinence period is also drug dependent, with longer abstinence periods occurring with drugs producing longer intake periods (e.g., d-amphetamine). Onset of a new drug-intake period is followed by responding at an initially high rate, quickly decreasing to a steady lower rate. Throughout the remainder of the session interresponse times gradually lengthen. Following several hours of drug abstinence, a new intake period can be initiated by delivering a single forced drug injection (a "prime"). The lengths of the drug-intake and abstinence periods do not seem to be related to the length of the preceding period or time of day, although the latter may be a factor in the self-administration of other stimulants, as shall be seen later.

Occasionally, if several drug injections occur close together, the animal may go on a drug "binge," with responding at a high rate and drug injections taken one after another until the injection system is shut off, or death occurs. Several thousands of responses often occur during such binges. These binges rarely occur, being most likely immediately after surgery when the animal is still partially under the effects of pentobarbital anesthesia, or when the drug is suddenly returned following a brief extinction period while the animal is responding at a high rate. The latter typically occurs when the infusion pump syringe sometimes unknowingly runs empty, and is not refilled for a short time. Such binges have now been almost completely eliminated by using the much briefer acting methoxyflurane gas anesthesia and continuous-reservoir infusion pumps.

During drug-intake periods the animals are highly excitable, do not eat or sleep, and exhibit highly stereotyped movements. The latter consist of rapid up and down, or right and left, head movements, and face-washing motions. The magnitude of these responses is greater with the higher drug doses. Under very high doses, chewing of the front feet and leg hair, and dysfunction of the lower extremities sometimes occur. With methamphetamine self-administration, occasional prolonged periods of penile erection accompanied by chewing of the hair around the genital area are also seen. During drug abstinence periods the animals sleep and eat.

The relatively long interresponse intervals characterizing stimulant self-administration might appear to be explained by temporary drug satiation resulting from each drug injection. However, since intravenously injected cocaine also produces a dose-related interruption in responding by rats on a FR food-reinforced baseline (Pickens and Thompson, 1968), it is possible that the long interresponse intervals observed in cocaine reinforcement is due, at least partly, to a more general behavior-disrupting effect of the drug. While this may be the case, it is important to note that the pause in FR food-reinforced responding could also be explained by the anorexigenic effects of the drug, making the animal effectively food satiated. That cocaine does not produce a complete behavioral disruption is indicated by the initially increased activity elicited by drug injections, and also by the drug "binges," where animals are capable of responding through a series of several successive drug injections.

CHRONIC DRUG EFFECTS

Over the course of several drug-intake periods, progressive changes occur in body weight and activity level. For animals receiving methamphetamine, weight losses up to 35 to 40 percent are sometimes observed after several weeks of self-administration. For animals receiving cocaine, however, weight loss of only 5 to 10 percent is typical, although this drug is also reputed to be a powerful appetite suppressant (Jaffe, 1965). Perhaps the difference is due to cocaine's very rapid metabolism, whereas methamphetamine is metabolized more slowly. During drug abstinence periods, cocaine animals would therefore recover more rapidly from the drug's anorexic effects, allowing them to regain more weight than the methamphetamine animals. The early death of the methamphetamine animals commonly occurring after three to

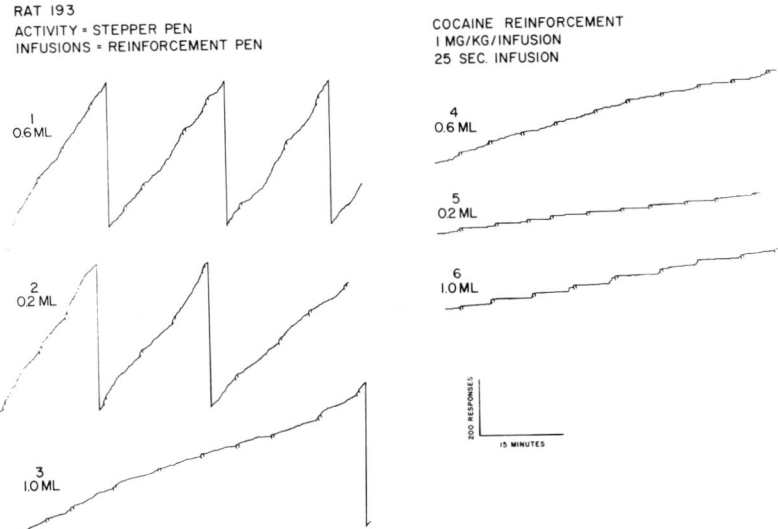

Fig. 3. Activity changes during cocaine reinforcement. Activity recorded by an ultrasonic motion detector operated by the stepper pen of the cumulative recorder, and cocaine infusions are indicated by downward deflections of the reinforcement pen.

four weeks of self-administration may be related to their large weight loss. Cocaine animals tend to live much longer. For the methamphetamine animals, however, when drug access is limited to 12 hours per day, the periods of drug intake occur only within the experimental session. Under these conditions no further abstinence periods occur, with the drug-intake periods elicited at the start of an experimental session by a drug "prime." Weight loss is greatly reduced by such a schedule.

Changes in activity over successive drug-intake sessions is apparently not related to weight loss. Initially, activity is high immediately after each injection and decreases slightly before the next. However, over several drug-intake periods, activity elicited by drug injection gradually decreases, while that occurring just before injection increases. Eventually, activity is no longer produced by drug injection, with activity increase observed only before each injection, as shown in Figure 3. That this activity is not the cause of the drug injection is indicated by the fact that no responding is seen during this time on a second cage lever which is a control lever, having no programmed consequence. The new activity pattern is evident at the start of each drug-intake period, and cannot be due to accumulation of drug and possible toxic effects. While the gradual decrease in activity elicited by drug injections may reflect drug tolerance, this change also occurs with drugs for which physiologic tolerance has never before been reported (Jaffe, 1965). Thus, while it is possible that tolerance occurs to these drugs under the present conditions, it is more likely that the effect is related to drug reinforcement-activity interactions (Pickens, Dougherty, and Thompson, 1969).

EXPERIMENTAL CONTROLS

Because stimulants are self-administered by rats does not necessarily mean that the drugs are serving as reinforcers. The self-administration behavior might be explained by some other drug effects. Several control experiments have demonstrated that stimulant self-administration is controlled by its consequences, and is therefore a drug-reinforcement effect. During a drug-intake period, if saline is substituted for the drug solution, or if drug injections are discontinued, extinction-like effects occur, with an initially high response rate decreasing gradually over time. If the cage contains two response levers, one of which delivers the drug injection and the other has no effect, responding occurs only on the drug lever. However, if these lever functions are reversed, the lever preference also reverses. Discontinuing the light paired with drug injections has essentially no effect on the behavior. If noncontingent drug injections are given, with an inter-injection interval equal

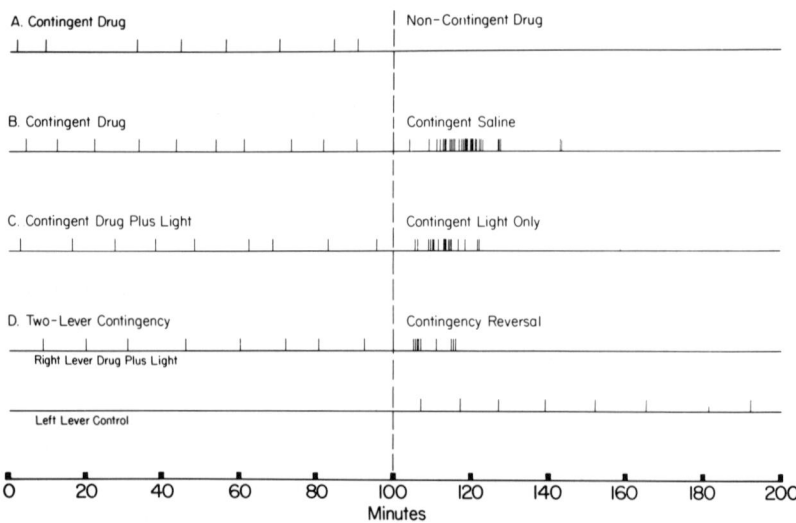

Fig. 4. Effects of various manipulations on responding for cocaine reinforcement. See text for explanation of procedures. (From Pickens and Thompson. J. Pharmacol. Exp. Ther. 1968, 161, 122-129. Courtesy of The Williams & Wilkins Co., Baltimore, Maryland.)

to the mean drug self-administration interval, and this schedule is superimposed on an existing self-administration schedule, no further self-administration responding occurs. Responding is resumed, however, when the noncontingent injections are discontinued (Fig. 4). Finally, if animals are paired and the experimental member of each pair is allowed to self-administer a low drug dose, while the control (yoked) member is given a drug injection at the same time as its experimental partner, the response rate of the experimental animal will be significantly above that of the control. These results indicate that response-contingent drug administration controls behavior in a manner similar to that of other consequences controlling responding, indicating these drugs are serving as reinforcers (Pickens and Thompson, 1968; Pickens, Meisch, and McGuire, 1967).

STIMULANT REINFORCEMENT IN OTHER ANIMALS

Alternating periods of stimulant intake and abstinence have also been reported for the monkey and human. Deneau, Yanagita, and Seevers (1964) described periods of cocaine and d-amphetamine self-administration by monkeys lasting for more than three days, followed by drug abstinence periods lasting from one to two days. Restlessness, stereotyped movements, weight loss, and biting of the extremities were commonly exhibited by these animals. During drug abstinence periods the monkeys slept for the first few hours, and then returned to seemingly normal behavior before the start of the next drug-intake period. Similar periods of drug intake and abstinence have also been reported for SPA and fencamfamine self-administration by monkeys (Estrada, Villarreal, and Schuster, 1967). Wilson, Hitomi, and Schuster (1969) have recently found response "patterning" to occur during methylphenidate self-administration by monkeys, with the length of the interresponse interval being dose dependent.

Behavioral patterns strikingly similar to those of the rat and monkey have also been seen with intravenous stimulant self-administration by humans. Kramer, Fischman, and Littlefield (1967) reported that in intravenous methamphetamine self-administration by humans, the drug is typically injected about every two hours around the clock for periods of three to six days, during which the individual remains awake continuously, eats little food, engages in stereotyped behavior, and becomes increasingly paranoid. Sometimes the drug-intake periods continue for as many as 12 days. The drug abstinence periods, which follow, are characterized initially by sleeping and eating, and later by decreased activity. During this time there is a gradual decrease in the paranoid state. Although no indication of the length of these abstinence periods was given, they may last several days, and conform to some extent to environmental demands, as would be the case in the weekend drug user (Griffith, 1966).

These data suggest that the lengths of drug-intake and abstinence periods increase as the phylogenetic scale is ascended from rat to monkey to man. The general characteristics of the stimulant drug reinforcement, however, do not change.

COMPARISON OF INTRAVENOUS AND INHALATION METHODS OF STIMULANT REINFORCEMENT

Deneau and Inoki (1967), using monkeys, studied the self-administration of nicotine by intravenous injection, and Jarvik (1967) studied the same behavior in the same animals, but using drug self-administration by inhalation. While a comparison of the findings of these two studies would be interesting, it is confounded by the fact that Deneau and Inoki used solutions of nicotine alkaloid dissolved in saline, whereas Jarvik used burning tobacco which contains not only nicotine but other substances as well. Nevertheless, remarkable behavioral similarities were reported in the two studies. Of particular importance is that alternating periods of nicotine intake and abstinence were found in both studies, indicating that this stimulant reinforcement characteristic is not an artefact of the route of drug self-administration. The abstinence periods in the two studies occur at night, with drug intake returning the next morning. This apparent control of nicotine self-administration by day-night factors has not been observed with other stimulant drugs, suggesting that this may be a unique characteristic of nicotine. In neither study is sufficient information presented to indicate whether response patterning for nicotine self-administration occurs.

VARIABLES AFFECTING STIMULANT REINFORCEMENT

Deneau and Inoki (1967) with nicotine, and Deaneau, Yanagita and Seevers (1964) with cocaine and d-amphetamine, found the onset of stimulant self-administration by monkeys is controlled to some extent by dose (reinforcement magnitude). Unless the dose is above some minimum level, self-administration does not occur. The behavior can also be brought under the control of discriminative stimuli, with self-administration occurring only when a stimulus light is illuminated (Deneau, personal communication).

Response rate for stimulant self-administration is inversely related to

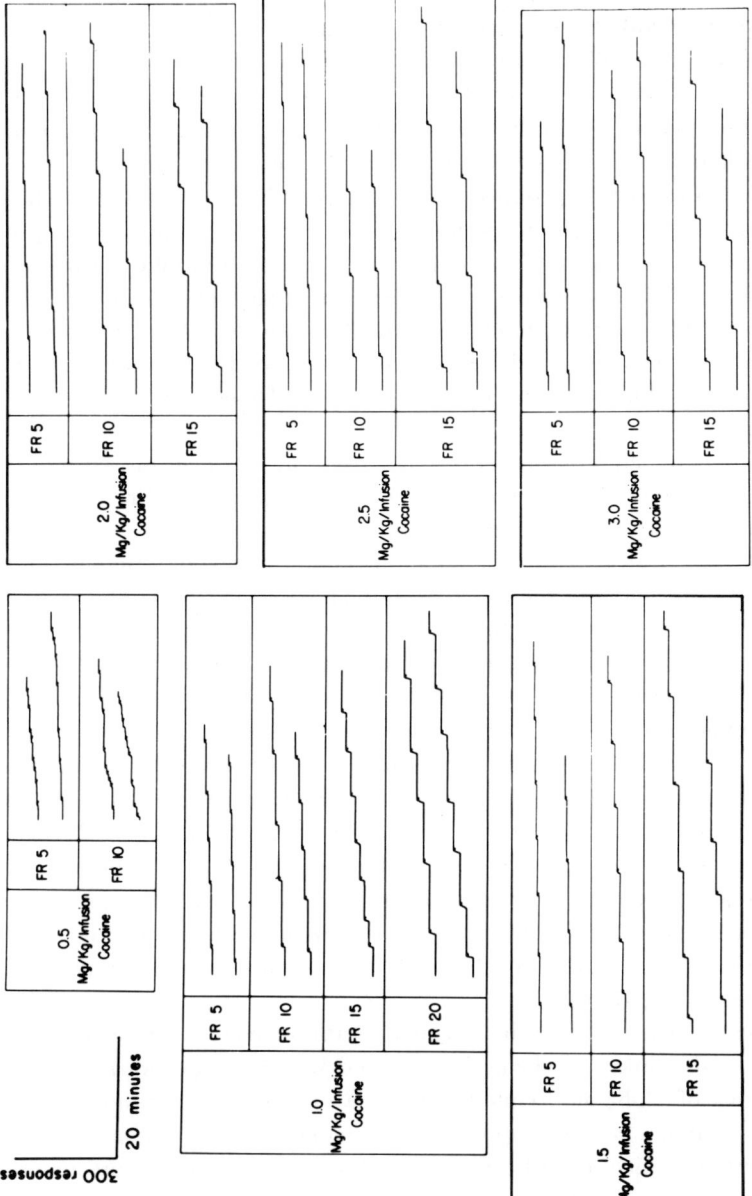

Fig. 5. Cumulative records of fixed-ratio cocaine self-administration in the rat at all doses and ratios which maintained responding for this subject.

187

dose (Pickens, 1968; Woods and Schuster, 1968). Responding for d-amphetamine (Pickens and Thompson, 1967; Pickens and Harris, 1968), methamphetamine (Pickens, Meisch, and McGuire, 1967), and cocaine (Pickens and Thompson, 1968) by rats, and fencamfamin and SPA (Estrada, Villarreal, and Schuster, 1967), methylphenidate, pipradrol, phenmetrazine (Wilson, Hitomi, and Schuster, 1969) by monkeys, decreases with increases in drug dose, and increases with decreases in dose. Thus, the total hourly amount of drug taken at each dose per injection is essentially the same. Very low cocaine doses in rats produce irregular responding, at times extinction-like effects, and very high doses produce an abrupt cessation of responding (Pickens and Thompson, 1968). The same is true in monkeys with nicotine (Deneau and Inoki, 1967) and other stimulants (Schuster, Woods, and Seevers, 1968). Variations in injection duration (length) and volume (drug concentration), with dose held constant, have no effect on the frequency of cocaine self-administration by rats (Pickens, Dougherty, and Thompson, 1969).

Stimulant self-administration has been maintained on several simple intermittent reinforcement schedules. Rats respond on FR schedules for self-administration of d-amphetamine (Pickens and Thompson, 1967; Pickens and Harris, 1968), methamphetamine (Pickens, Meisch, and McGuire, 1968), and cocaine (Pickens and Thompson, 1967). The characteristics of this schedule performance are shown in Figure 5. The behavior pattern generated by FR cocaine reinforcement is similar to that seen with other reinforcers, except a much longer post-reinforcement pause occurs. Drug intake remains essentially constant across all ratio values, and somewhat higher FR values can be maintained with intermediate cocaine doses than with either lower or higher doses (Pickens and Thompson, 1968). Monkeys have been maintained on FI (Figure 6) and VI (Figure 7) schedules for cocaine reinforcement. On both of these schedules, responding is similar to that maintained by other reinforcers. Terminal response rate on FI schedules for cocaine reinforcement increases with increases in drug dose and decreases in FI value. On VI schedules, response rate also increases with increases in drug dose.

Chemical interactions in stimulant reinforcement have been studied in the rat and monkey. Pickens, Meisch, and Dougherty (1968b) reported that injections of alpha-methylparatyrosine, a depleter of brain norepinephrine, and methamphetamine, suppress methamphetamine self-administration by rats, but that injections of L-dopa, which is a norepinephrine precursor, have no effect. Wilson and Schuster (1968) found responding for cocaine rein-

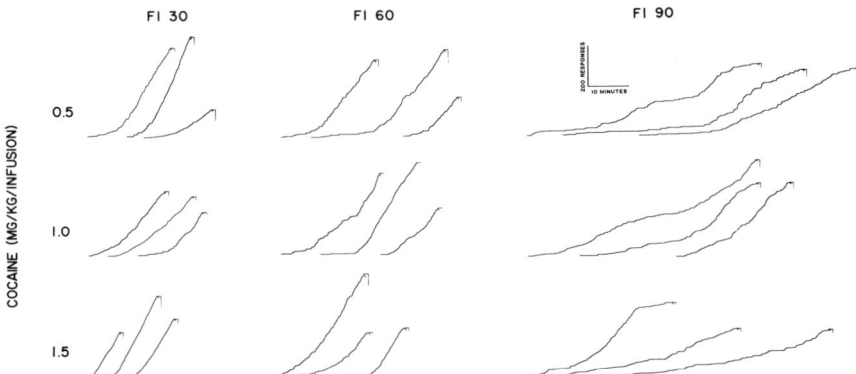

Fig. 6. Cumulative records of fixed-interval (30, 60, 90 min) cocaine reinforcement at 0.5, 1.0, and 1.5 mg/kg/infusion. Portions of each record before first response have been deleted to save space.

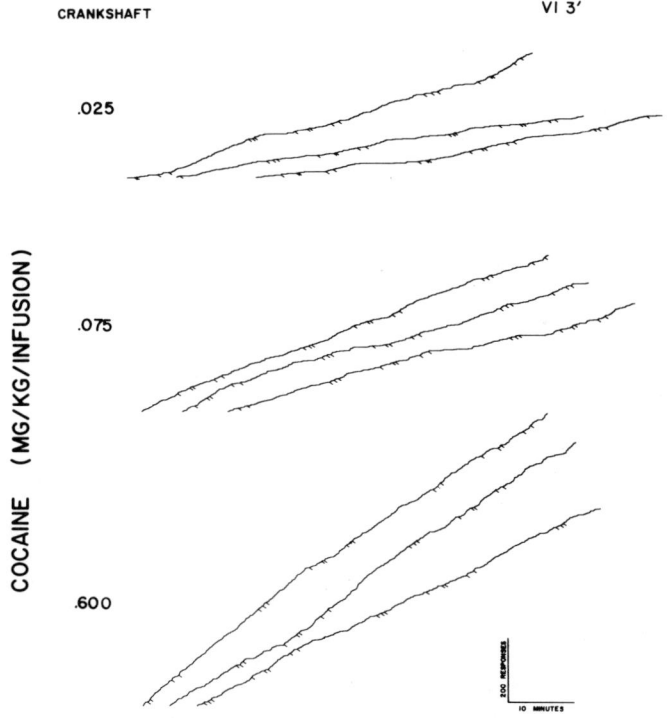

Fig. 7. Cumulative records of variable interval 3 min cocaine reinforcement at .025, .075, and .600 mg/kg/infusion.

forcement by monkeys increases following pretreatment with chlorpromazine and trifluoperazine, and that SPA reinforcement increases following chlorpromazine, but pentobarbital and morphine decrease the response rate for both drugs, and phenoxybenzamine and phentolamine have essentially no effect.

A CAUTIONARY NOTE

While it is obvious that the characteristics of stimulant drug reinforcement are in many ways similar to those of other reinforcers, differences also exist. It is possible that at least some differences can be explained on the basis of procedural factors. For example, cocaine reinforcement experiments may last up to 24 hours per day, whereas food reinforcement experiments are often much shorter. Some of the apparent differences between the behavior generated by these two reinforcers disappear when similar session lengths are used (Pickens and Thompson, 1968; Pickens, Bloom, and Thompson, 1969). Undoubtedly many more procedural factors may also account for some of the other differences between the effects of these reinforcers.

REFERENCES

Axelrod, J. Metabolism of epinephrine and of the sympathiomimetic amines. *Physiol. Rev.*, 1959, *39*, 751.

Davis, J.D. A method for chronic intravenous infusion in freely moving rats. *J. Exp. Anal. Behav.*, 1966, *9*, 385.

Deneau, G.A., and Inoki, R. Nicotine self-administration in monkeys. *Ann. N.Y. Acad. Sci.*, 1967, *142*, 277.

────── Yanagita, T., and Seevers, M.H. Self-administration of drugs by monkeys. Reported to the NAS-NRC Committee on Problems of Drug Dependence, 1964.

Eddy, N.B., Halback, H., Isbell, H., and Seevers, M.H. Drug dependence: Its significance and characteristics. *Bull. WHO*, 1965, *32*, 721.

Ellis, S. The metabolic effects of epinephrine and related amines. *Pharmacol. Rev.*, 1956, *8*, 485.

Estrada, U., Villarreal, J.E., and Schuster, C.R. Self-administration of stimulant drugs as a function of the dose per injection. Reported to the NAS-NRC Committee on Problems of Drug Dependence, 1967.

Goth, A. *Medical Pharmacology.* St. Louis, The C.V. Mosby Co., 1968.

Griffith, J. A study of illicit amphetamine drug traffic in Oklahoma City. *Amer. J. Psychiat.*, 1966, *123*, 560.

Jaffe, J.H. Drug addiction and drug abuse. In L.S. Foodman and A. Gilman, eds., *The Pharmacological Basis of Therapeutics.* New York, The Macmillan Company, 1965.

Jarvik, M.E. Tobacco smoking in monkeys. *Ann. N. Y. Acad. Sci.*, 1967, *142*, 280.

Kosman, M.E., and Unna, K.R. Effects of chronic administration of the amphetamines and other stimulants on behavior. *Clin. Pharmacol. Ther.*, 1968, *9*, 240.

Kramer, J.C., Fischman, V.S., and Littlefield, D.C. Amphetamine abuse. *JAMA*, 1967, *201*, 89.

Leake, C.D. *The Amphetamines: Their Actions and Uses.* Springfield, Ill., Charles C Thomas, Publisher, 1958.

McGuire, L.E. Reinforcing effects of intravenously-infused morphine and 1-methamphetamine. Unpublished doctoral dissertation. University of Mississippi, 1966.

Muscholl, E. Indirectly acting sympathomimetic amines. *Pharmacol. Rev.*, 1966, *18*, 551.

Pickens, R. Self-administration of stimulants by rats. *The International Journal of the Addictions*, 1968, *3*, 215.

—— and Harris, W.C. Self-administration of d-amphetamine by rats. *Psychopharmacologia*, 1968, *12*, 158.

—— and Thompson, T. Self-administration of amphetamine and cocaine by rats. Reported to the NAS-NRC Committee on Problems of Drug Dependence, 1967.

—— and Thompson, T. Cocaine-reinforced behavior in rats: Effects of reinforcement magnitude and fixed-ratio size. *J. Pharmacol. Exp. Ther.*, 1968, *161*, 122.

—— Bloom, W., and Thompson, T. Response rate as a function of long session lengths and large reinforcement magnitudes. Proceedings American Psychological Association, 1969, 809-810.

—— Dougherty, J.A., and Thompson, T. Effects of volume and duration of infusion on cocaine reinforcement, with concurrent activity recording. Reported to the NAS-NRC Committee on Problems of Drug Dependence, 1969.

—— Meisch, R.A., and Dougherty, J.A. Effects of behavioral and biochemical manipulations on methamphetamine self-administration in the rat. Reported to the NAS-NRC Committee on Problems of Drug Dependence, 1968a.

—— Meisch, R.A., and Dougherty, J.A. Chemical interactions in methamphetamine reinforcement. *Psychol. Rep.*, 1968(b), *23*, 1267.

—— Meisch, R., and McGuire, L.E. Methamphetamine reinforcement in rats. *Psychonomic Science*, 1967, *8*, 371.

Schuster, C.R., Woods, J.H., and Seevers, M.H. Self-administration of central stimulants by the monkey. Presented at Symposium on Abuse of Central Stimulants, Karolinska Institute, Stockholm, Sweden, 1968.

Seevers, M.H. and Deneau, G.A. Physiological aspects of tolerance and physical dependence. In W.S. Root and F.G. Hofmann, eds., *Physiological Pharmacology.* Volume I. New York, Academic Press, Inc., 1963, 565.

Thompson, T., and Pickens, R. Drug self-administration and conditioning. In H. Steinberg, ed., *Scientific Basis of Drug Dependence.* London, J. & A. Churchill, Ltd., 1968.

—— and Pickens, R. Behavioral variables influencing drug self-administration. In R.T. Harris, W.M. McIsaac, and C.R. Schuster, eds., *Drug Dependence.* Austin, University of Texas Press, 1970.

Weiss, B., and Laties, V.G. Enhancement of human performance by caffeine and the amphetamines. *Pharmacol. Rev.*, 1962, *14*, 1.

Wilson, M.C., and Schuster, C.R. Pharmacological modification of the self-administration of cocaine and SPA in the rhesus monkey. Reported to the NAS-NRC Committee on Problems of Drug Dependence, 1968.

—— Hitomi, M., and Schuster, C.R. Further studies of the self-administration of psychomotor stimulants in the rhesus monkey. Reported to the Committee on Problems of Drug Dependence, 1969.

Woods, J.H., and Schuster, C.R. Reinforcement properties of morphine, cocaine, and SPA as a function of unit dose. *The International Journal of the Addictions*, 1968, *3*, 231.

Yanagita, T., Deneau, G.A., and Seevers, M.H. Evaluation of pharmacologic agents in the monkey by long term intravenous self or programmed administration. *Excerpta Medica International Congress Series*, 1965, *87*, 453.

12
Environmental Variables Influencing Drug Self-Administration[1]

Travis Thompson, George Bigelow, and Roy Pickens[2]

Departments of Psychiatry and Pharmacology
University of Minnesota
Minneapolis, Minnesota

Behavioral effects of drugs depend not only on their direct pharmacologic actions, but on the contingencies maintaining behavior as well (Sidman, 1956). This notion of drug-environment interaction applies equally to the analysis of factors influencing drug self-administration (Thompson and Schuster, 1968). Whether a drug will be self-administered depends not only on the type of drug, but also on the environmental conditions under which the drug is made available. Among the classes of environmental variables determining whether a drug will be self-administered are (a) past history of the subjects, (b) motivational factors, (c) current environmental conditions, and (d) reinforcement variables (Schuster and Thompson, 1969).

PRIOR HISTORY

The prior history of subjects subsequently provided with the opportunity to self-administer drugs can be of two types: (1) the behavioral history and (2) prior experience with drugs (Thompson and Pickens, 1969).

Behavioral history. Weeks and Collins (1967) investigated the effect of behavioral history on subsequent tendency to self-administer morphine. One group of rats were conditioned to self-administer morphine by emitting a

---

[1] The research reported in this chapter was supported by Research Grants MH-15349, MH-14112, and MH-08565 from USPHS to the University of Minnesota.
[2] The authors are particularly grateful to R.A. Meisch for permitting us to present his data in this report.

lever-pressing response, while a control group received the same number and frequency of injections, but no response was required. After a period of detoxification, both groups were given the opportunity to self-administer morphine. Animals with previous experience emitting a response for morphine infusion learned the self-administration response significantly more rapidly than controls having learned no specific response for the drug.

Drug experience. Meisch and Pickens (1967) and Meisch (1969) illustrated the effect of prior drug experience on subsequent ethanol self-administration. The rate and volume of ethanol self-administered were compared during extinction of a previously food-reinforced response for subjects having a prior history of ethanol self-administration with those receiving only water. Rats were induced to orally self-administer ethanol and water using the schedule-induced polydipsia technique originally reported by Falk

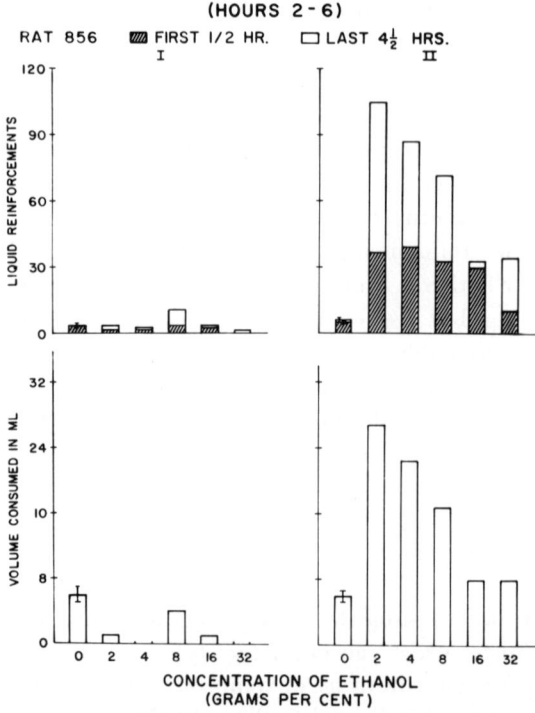

Fig. 1. The effects of ethanol experience on oral ethanol self-administration by a rat. I. The number of liquid reinforcements at 2 to 32 grams percent concentration and the volume of fluid ingested during extinction of a previously food-reinforced response. During food reinforcement, tap water had been available and copious drinking occurred adjunctively. II. After a history of ethanol consumption via schedule-induced polydipsia, there is a significant increase in the number of ethanol reinforcements (top graph) and the volume of ethanol consumed (bottom graph) (Meisch, unpublished).

(1961). Under such conditions, rats that are not water-deprived will drink up to 10 times their normal daily intake of water. Initially, rats were trained in the polydipsia situation until their daily water intake stabilized, then food reinforcement was discontinued. During food-extinction sessions, the only fluid available was ethanol, varying in concentration from 2 to 32 grams percent. Very little ethanol was consumed under these conditions (see the left side of Figure 1). However, when the polydipsia contingencies were reinstated and animals were exposed to ethanol every third day (8 grams percent), subsequent food-extinction produced a substantially increased ethanol consumption (right half of Figure 1).

MOTIVATIONAL CONDITIONS

Opiate deprivation and satiation. It has been suggested that animals physically dependent on morphine, self-administer the drug to escape from or avoid withdrawal distress (Nichols, 1957). While this is a plausible hypothesis, there is no direct evidence indicating this is necessarily the case. In fact some findings suggest morphine can serve as a reinforcer at doses which do not produce physical dependence (Woods and Schuster, 1968), indicating that such animals cannot be responding to avoid withdrawal. The motivating influence of morphine deprivation in physically dependent animals has been reported by several investigators. Monkeys increased their rate of responding in both components of an FI-FR chained schedule of morphine reinforcement (Thompson and Schuster, 1964). Wikler et al. (1963) reported that rats made physically dependent on opiates by daily morphine injections, when deprived of the drug for varying periods, showed an orderly increase in consumption of an etonitazine (synthetic opioid) solution over tap water. Morphine deprivation can also be induced chemically, e.g., by administering the antagonist nalorphine. Weeks (1962) found that 4 mg/kg i.p. of nalorphine caused the rate of morphine self-administration to increase, and Thompson and Schuster (1964) reported similar effects in monkeys. Weeks and Collins (1964) reported that etonitazine introduced into the drinking water reduced morphine-reinforced lever pressing, apparently by a satiation effect. Thompson and Pickens (1969) reported that hourly i.m. injections of the synthetic opioid, methadone, reduced morphine-reinforced FR 30 performance, proportional to dose of methadone (Fig. 2).

In the studies outline above, deprivation was imposed by the experimenter. Thompson, Bigelow and Pickens (1969) conditioned monkeys to engage in a complex response sequence, providing one monkey with an opportunity to obtain morphine intravenously, and a paired monkey to

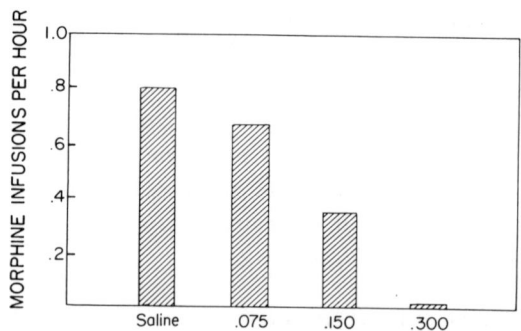

Fig. 2. The effect of hourly intramuscular injections of methadone on the number of morphine self-administrations per hour on a Fixed-Ratio 30 schedule by a physically dependent rhesus monkey. There is an inverse relation between the dose of methadone and the rate of morphine self-administration (Thompson and Pickens, 1969).

obtain food, water or apricots. In order for either monkey to obtain its respective reinforcers, cooperative behavior was required. The degree to which the animals engaged in cooperative behavior determined the period of morphine deprivation. A large sample of behavior was obtained over several months representing a range of periods of socially imposed morphine deprivation. Figure 3 shows the effect of the degree of cooperativeness of the two monkeys (expressed as minutes of morphine deprivation) on the time to complete 75 responses for a morphine infusion, once the opportunity was provided. At deprivation periods longer than 400 minutes, there was a marked shift toward short times to complete the FR-75 requirement, while at deprivation periods less than 200 minutes, there were many longer times.

Motivational manipulations with stimulants. Studies of stimulant drug deprivation have not been reported at this writing. An apparent motivational effect has been observed with self-administration of stimulants paralleling observations with intracranial self-stimulation. Following a period of forced drug abstinence, rats will frequently not initiate self-administration for some time after being placed in the experimental chamber. If, however, a free infusion is given at the beginning of the session, self-administration is generally initiated within 10 to 15 minutes (i.e., approximately the inter-self-infusion interval). A similar "priming" effect has been observed with self-stimulation of the brain, and has been interpreted as a motivational effect (Olds, 1962).

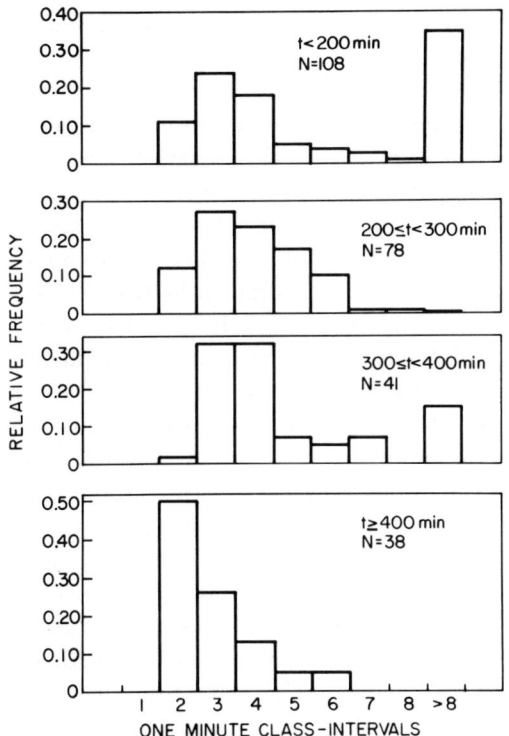

Fig. 3. The effect of socially imposed morphine deprivation on the time to complete a Fixed Ratio of 75, for intravenous morphine in the rhesus monkey. The relative frequency of latencies from 1 to 8 minutes or longer are shown for deprivation times of less than 200 minutes (top graph), to greater than 400 minutes (bottom graph). Deprivation time was determined by the degree to which two monkeys cooperated to have access to respective reinforcers (Thompson, Bigelow, and Pickens, 1969).

CURRENT ENVIRONMENTAL CONDITIONS

Environmental "stress." Davis and Miller (1963) and Davis, Lulenski and Miller (1968) reported that noncontingent foot shock induced barbiturate self-administration by rats. Kamano and Arp (1965) failed to find such an effect in an effort to induce rats to drink chlordiazepoxide. Masserman and Yum (1946) reported that cats in a "conflict" situation consumed ethanol, and Clark and Polish (1960) found monkeys increased ethanol consumption when they were placed on a shock avoidance schedule. Mello and Mendelson (1964) demonstrated that shock avoidance schedules evoked an abrupt increase in alcohol consumption in a monkey which freely selected alcohol prior to conditioning.

Stimulus generalization. In addition to inducing nondependent rats to self-administer drugs, the similarity of environmental conditions during self-administration to those in which the behavior was originally established appears to be of importance. Thompson and Ostlund (1964) made rats physically dependent on morphine using an oral administration procedure similar to that described by Nichols, Headlee and Coppock (1956). For 30 days of morphine deprivation (withdrawal) half of the rats were moved to a markedly different environment and half were left in the original environment. Following withdrawal there was a readdiction phase during which half of each group remained in the withdrawal environment and the other half was moved to the other original environment. During this three-week readdiction phase, oral preference tests were run to assess relative disposition to ingest morphine solutions. Animals returned to the same environments in which original drug administration had occurred ingested significantly larger amounts of morphine, and animals placed in an environment different from that in which withdrawal had occurred ingested relatively great amounts of morphine. That is, the tendency to self-administer is greater if the environment is the same as that in which the original drug-taking had occurred and, conversely, placing the animal in the situation where withdrawal has occurred decreased the probability of drug self-administration.

The social environment. Little research has dealt with the role of social variables in drug self-administration. In an effort to explore the role of basic social interdependencies, Thompson, Bigelow and Pickens (1969) designed a multi-compartment experimental space where free-moving monkeys obtained several reinforcers, including morphine. Figure 4 shows two monkeys in adjacent compartments, one responding for food and the paired animal about to respond for morphine.

Subjects worked in pairs, one to obtain food, water, and fruit under visual stimulus control in one compartment of the chamber, and the other to self-administer morphine via a radio-controlled infusion pump under visual stimulus control in another compartment. The terminal behavior sequence leading to food, water, and fruit reinforcement included: (1) Standing on a platform scale immediately outside the food, water, and fruit compartment in the presence of an appropriate stimulus light. When the correct animal stood on the scale (as determined by his weight), a solenoid lock would release and the animal could open the door and enter the work compart-

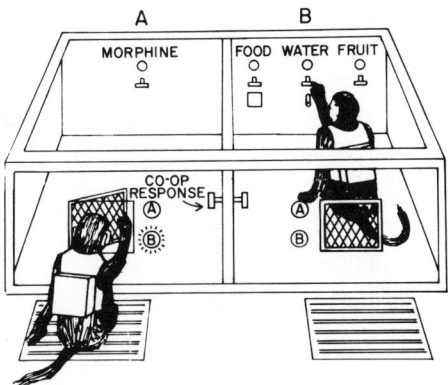

Fig. 4. Drawing of two monkeys in adjacent compartments in a complex social experiment in which morphine is self-administered. Monkeys are equipped with leather vests supporting a backpack containing a radio-controlled infusion pump. Monkey A is about to enter the compartment where he will be provided with the opportunity to self-administer morphine intravenously, and Monkey B is responding on the water lever in a three member nonreversible option (Thompson, Bigelow, and Pickens, 1969).

ment. (2) When the door was opened and closed, a "cooperative" stimulus light was illuminated on the screen panel separating this compartment from the adjacent morphine compartment. (3) If the monkeys in the two adjacent compartments concurrently held their respective toggle switches closed for a specified interval, the stimulus lights over the food, water, and fruit levers would be illuminated. (4) The monkey could then proceed to respond to obtain these reinforcers by operating each lever a fixed number of times. This session lasted for a fixed time period after which the lights were extinguished. (5) Operation of a pushbutton alongside the compartment door allowed the animal to re-enter the large cage social area at the end of the work session. The program then recycled.

The terminal behavior sequence leading to morphine reinforcement was comparable. Entrance to and exit from the morphine compartment were controlled in the same manner as for the food compartment. The consequence of completing the cooperative response requirement was illumination of the stimulus light for the drug self-administration lever. A fixed number of responses on this lever produced morphine infusion, during which the stimulus light flashed. Only one drug infusion was permitted during each session.

During some portions of the experiment, these two behavioral sequences were combined as shown in Figure 5. In this sequence, once the food mon-

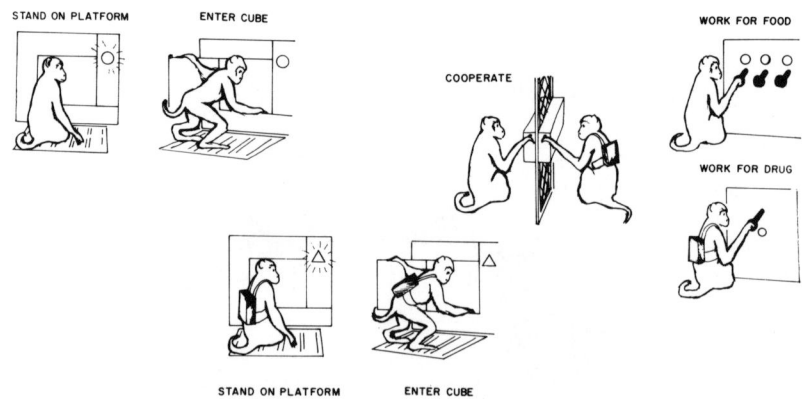

Fig. 5. Behavioral sequence for two monkeys in which one monkey works to obtain access to food, water, and fruit (top animal) and another works to have access to the opportunity to self-administer morphine (bottom). The contingencies of the sequence are described in text, and proceed from left to right (Thompson, Bigelow, and Pickens, 1969).

key had entered his compartment, the stimulus light on the door to the morphine compartment was illuminated to allow the drug monkey to enter his compartment. Once both compartments were occupied, the two animals could cooperate and then respond for their respective reinforcers. This combined behavior sequence was designed for eventual expansion to a three-monkey situation in which each animal would have the opportunity to self-administer morphine and work for his food, water, and fruit. Pairing arrangement could be established such that for each monkey each class of reinforcers was uniquely paired with a different animal.

Figure 6 shows cumulative records of responding for food (FR 75), apricots (FR 30), and water (FR 20) by one monkey, and FR 75 performance by a paired monkey for 4.75 mg/kg of morphine during three successive periods (A, B, and C) spaced two hours apart. The top events record shows the intervals during which depression of the cooperative toggle switch by both monkeys would illuminate their respective work lights associated with food, water, fruit, and morphine reinforcement. The second and third events records indicate the responses made by the two monkeys on their cooperation switches. The drug monkey depressed his switch and held it down, while the food monkey more erratically opened and closed his switch. The fixed-ratio performance for the ingestive reinforcers is typical, with occasional grainy performance and strain (Ferster and Skinner, 1957), while the FR performance of the paired morphine monkey is much more irregular.

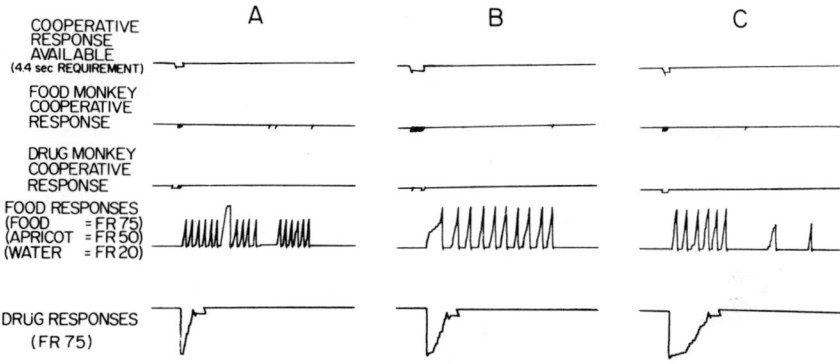

Fig. 6. Sample concurrent records of performance by paired animals responding for food, water, and apricots (upper cumulative record) or morphine (lower cumulative record). The top events pen is deflected when the cooperative switch holding response will be reinforced, and the second and third events pens show responses on the cooperative switch by the food and drug monkeys, respectively (Thompson, Bigelow, and Pickens, 1969).

Nonetheless, the "break-and-run" feature characteristic of fixed ratio performance for any reinforcer on an FR schedule is apparent.

The degree to which it was possible to establish and maintain cooperative

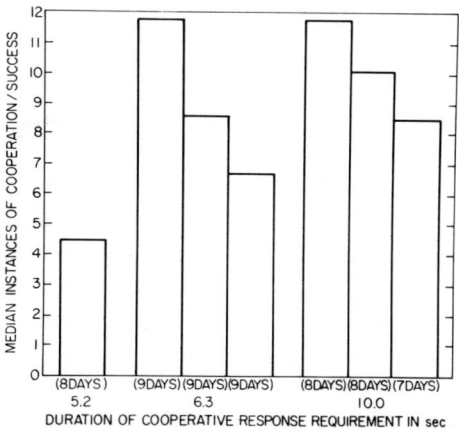

Fig. 7. Efficiency of the cooperative switch holding response as a function of the duration with which the cooperative switches must be held closed. The number of days each value was in effect is indicated below successive columns. With increasing durations, the efficiency decreased (i.e., the instances of cooperation per successful cooperation increased), but with exposure the contingencies performance progressively improved (Thompson, Bigelow, and Pickens, 1969).

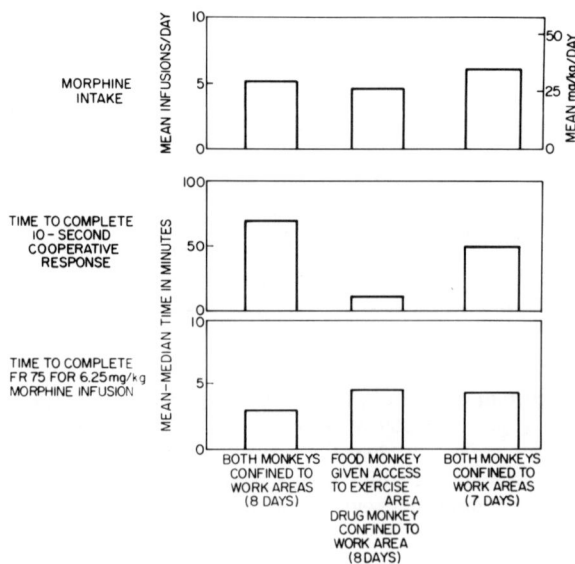

Fig. 8. The effect of restricting access of one monkey on morphine self-administration performance of the paired monkey. The time to complete the cooperative response decreased and the time to complete the FR 75 increased, when the food monkey was allowed free movement but the morphine monkey was restricted to its work compartment (Thompson, Bigelow, and Pickens, 1969).

switch-holding for access to morphine, or food, water, and fruit, is shown in Figure 7. For eight days, both switches had to be held closed simultaneously for 5.2 seconds, and the median instances of attempts to cooperate relative to the number of successes was 4.5. The duration of the response requirement was increased to 6.3 seconds for 27 days. Initially, many more attempts to cooperate per success were observed, however, this ratio decreased substantially over 27 days. Increasing the duration of cooperation to 10 seconds produced a comparable decrement in cooperative efficiency, followed by gradual improvement, indicating progressive learning to tolerate longer cooperative requirements.

By confirming both animals to their work areas, the earlier members of the heterogeneous chain of responses leading to morphine self-administration were eliminated. Thus, only the cooperative response and the FR 75-morphine reinforced operants were required. Both monkeys were confined to their work areas for eight days, and morphine intake, time required to complete a 10-second cooperative response, and time to complete the FR 75 recorded. For the next eight days the food, water, and fruit monkey was allowed to leave and enter the outer social chamber, and the same dependent variables were recorded. Figure 8 shows that the time to complete the cooperative response decreased markedly when the food animal was allowed to move in and out freely, while the time for the morphine animal to complete the FR 75 for morphine increased substantially. The fact that the time to complete the cooperative response decreases suggests increased deprivation, however, this is rendered unlikely since the time to complete the FR 75 increases, which occurs under conditions of morphine satiation. Apparently the arrival of the food, water, and fruit monkey into the adjacent cubicle was a sufficient discriminative stimulus to set the occasion for the morphine monkey to complete the cooperative response even though he was not appreciably deprived of morphine at the time.

Concurrent reinforcement contingencies. Another class of current environmental conditions altering animals' disposition to self-administer drugs, are concurrent reinforcement schedules for other reinforcers. Drug self-administration via schedule-induced polydipsia was mentioned briefly above. Basically, this procedure consists of providing food reinforcement on a vari-

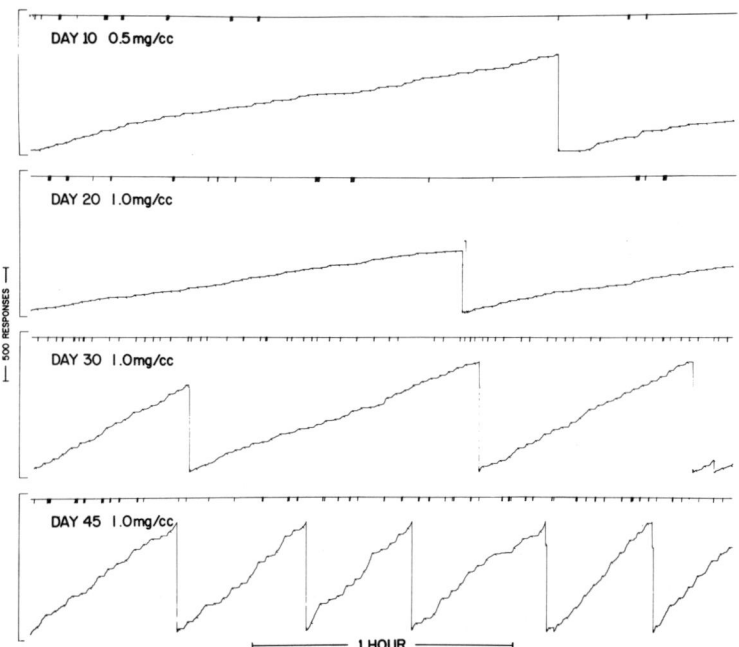

Fig. 9. Oral morphine self-administration by the rat via schedule-induced polydipsia. The cumulative recorder stepper pen shows food reinforced lever pressing on a fixed-interval two-minute schedule, while the events pen record above each cumulative record shows licks of the morphine solution using a drinkometer (Thompson, unpublished).

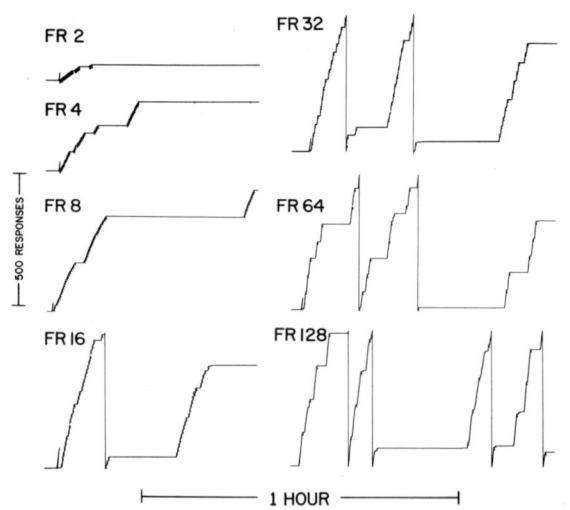

Fig. 10. Cumulative records of oral fixed-ratio ethanol self-administration by a rat after an extensive history of oral ethanol ingestion via schedule-induced polydipsia. Fixed-ratios ranging from FR 2 to FR 128 are shown in which ethanol concentration was held constant at 8 grams percent (Meisch and Thompson, unpublished).

able interval of one minute, and fluid reinforcement on a continuous schedule on a second lever. Figure 9 shows sample cumulative records of the development of polydipsia using morphine as the reinforcing drug. Initially, the concentration was 0.5 mg/ml, which was increased to 1.0 mg/ml after 14 days. At the end of 45 days, the animal was consuming from 80 to 100 ml of fluid (i.e., 80 to 100 mg orally) per day. The polydipsia method has also been used to induce consumption of pentobarbital (Meisch, 1969), with effects similar to earlier reports with polydipsia-induced self-administration of ethanol. Thus, the factors controlling ethanol self-administration cannot be due to caloric value of ethanol alone, since both morphine and pentobarbital, which have no caloric value produce similar patterns of oral self-administration. Figure 10 shows a sample cumulative record of FR 1 to FR 128 performance for ethanol after an extensive history of ethanol self-administration via polydipsia. Polydipsia was discontinued, and daily sessions run on which only ethanol was available. The degree to which good schedule control was exercised and the high response rates indicate ethanol was serving as an effective reinforcer. In each case, most of the ethanol was consumed during the first hour of the session, followed by approximately four hours without responding, terminating in another bout of ethanol-reinforced responding during the last hour of the session (Meisch and Thompson, unpublished).

REINFORCEMENT VARIABLES

The role of the type of drug reinforcer, the magnitude of reinforcement, duration, and volume of reinforcement, as well as simple schedules of drug reinforcement, have been reviewed elsewhere, and will not be discussed here (Thompson and Pickens, 1969; Schuster and Thompson, 1969).

Feedback stimuli. Among other significant reinforcement variables are stimulus conditions paired with drug infusion. It has been commonly observed that operant responses are learned more readily when feedback is provided immediately contingent on the response (Bugelski, 1938; Skinner, 1938, 1951). This is particularly true of drug reinforcement, where a considerable period elapses between the response until a significant amount of the reinforcing drug in the bloodstream (Pickens and Thompson, 1968).

It has also been shown that feedback stimuli can have discriminative stimulus functions (Holz and Azrin, 1961, 1962). Most recently Hake and Azrin (1969) found that responding is reduced during a feedback stimulus associated with food reinforcement. In drug self-administration studies, particularly those involving stimulant drugs, a prominent feature is absence of responding following the reinforced response. In addition to the direct suppressing effect of drug administration on further responding, another mechanism for this effect may relate to the rate-reducing effect of feedback stimuli. The consequence of a self-administration response is presumably a progressive interoceptive stimulus change produced by the drug, which also reinforces the antecedent behavior. Such interoceptive stimulus changes may have the functional status of rate-suppressing feedback stimuli.

Conditioned reinforcement. Stimuli paired with reinforcing drugs can also serve as reinforcers in their own right. Thompson and Schuster (1964) found that monkeys continued emitting an FI-FR chain of responses for up to 60 days following discontinuation of morphine reinforcement, when the only consequence was illumination of a light previously paired with morphine. Schuster and Woods (1967) observed a similar phenomenon, in which monkeys were presented with a light previously paired with morphine on a variable interval schedule, during alternate days of extinction. On days that the light was presented, significantly more responses were emitted than on alternate days when there were no programmed consequences following responding.

REFERENCES

Bugelski, R. Extinction with and without sub-goal reinforcement. *J. Comp. Physiol. Psychol.*, 1938, *26*, 121.

Clark, R., and Polish, E. Avoidance conditioning and alcohol consumption on rhesus monkeys. *Science*, 1960, *132*, 223.

Davis, J.D., and Miller, N.E. Fear and pain: Their effect on self-injection of amobarbital sodium by rats. *Science*, 1963, *141*, 1286.

──── Lulenski, G.C., and Miller, N.E. Comparative studies of barbiturate self-administration. *International Journal of the Addictions*, 1968, *3*, 207.

Falk, J.L. The production of polydipsia in normal rats by an intermittent food schedule. *Science*, 1961, *133*, 195.

Hake, D.F., and Azrin, N.H. A response-spacing effect: An absence of responding during response-feedback stimuli. *J. Exp. Anal. Behav.*, 1969, *12*, 17.

Holz, W.C., and Azrin, N.H. Discrimination properties of punishment. *J. Exp. Anal. Behav.*, 1961, *4*, 225.

──── and Azrin, N.H. Interactions between the discriminative and aversive properties of punishment. *J. Exp. Anal. Behav.*, 1962, *5*, 229.

Kamano, D.K., and Arp, D.J. Chlordiazepoxide (Librium) consumption under stress conditions in rats. *Int. J. Neuropsychiat.*, 1965, *1*, 189.

Masserman, J.H., and Yum, K.S. An analysis of the influence of alcohol on experimental neurosis in cats. *Psychosom. Med.*, 1946, *8*, 36.

Meisch, R.A. Self-administration of pentobarbital via schedule-induced polydipsia. *Psychonomic Science*, 1969, *16*, 16.

──── Increased Rate of Ethanol Self-Administration as a Function of Experience. (In press)

──── and Pickens, R. A new technique for oral self-administration of drugs by animals. Reported to the NAS-NRC Committee on Problems of Drug Dependence. February, 1968.

──── and Thompson, T. Fixed-ratio schedules of ethanol self-administration by rats. (Unpublished)

Mello, N.K., and Mendelson, J. Operant performance by rats for alcohol reinforcement. *Quart. J. Stud. Alcohol*, 1964, *25*, 226.

Nichols, J.R., Headlee, C.P., and Coppock, H.W. Drug addiction I. Addiction by escape training. *Journal of the American Pharmaceutical Association*, 1956, *45*, 788.

Olds, J. Hypothalamic substrate of reward. *Physiol. Rev.*, 1962, *42*, 554.

Schuster, C.R., and Thompson, T. Self-administration of and behavioral dependence on drugs. *Ann. Rev. Pharmacol.*, 1969, *9*, 483.

──── and Woods, J.A. The conditioned reinforcing effects of stimuli associated with morphine reinforcement. *International Journal of the Addictions*, 1968, *3*, 223.

Sidman, M. Drug behavior interaction. *Ann. N.Y. Acad. Sci.*, 1956, *65*, 282.

Skinner, B.F. *Behavior of Organisms.* New York, Appleton-Century-Crofts, 1938.

──── How to teach animals. *Sci. Amer.*, 1951, *185*, 26.

Thompson, T., Bigelow, G., and Pickens, R. Morphine self-administration by unrestrained monkeys in a complex programmed environment. Reported to the NAS-NRC Committee on Problems of Drug Dependence, Palo Alto, California, 1969.

──── and Ostlund, W. Susceptability to readdiction as a function of the addiction and withdrawal environment. *J. Comp. Physiol. Psychol.*, 1965, *59*, 388.

──── and Pickens, R. Drug self-administration and conditioning. In H. Steinberg, ed., *Scientific Basis of Drug Dependence*, London, J. & A. Churchill Ltd., 1969.

―― and Schuster, C.R. Morphine self-administration, food-reinforced and avoidance behaviors in rhesus monkeys. *Psychopharmacologia*, 1964, *5*, 87.

―― and Schuster, C.R. *Behavioral Pharmacology*. Englewood Cliffs, New Jersey, Prentice-Hall, Inc., 1968.

Weeks, J.R. Experimental morphine addiction: Method for automatic intravenous injection in unrestrained rats. *Science*, 1962, *138*, 143.

―― and Collins, R.J. Factors effecting voluntary morphine intake in self-maintained addicted rats. *Psychopharmacologia*, 1964, *6*, 267.

Wikler, A., Martin, W.R., Pescor, F.T., and Endes, C.G. Factors regulating oral consumption of an opioid (etonitazene) by morphine-addicted rats. *Psychopharmacologia*, 1963, *5*, 55-78.

Woods, J.H., and Schuster, C.R. Reinforcement properties of morphine, cocaine, and SPA as a function of unit dose. *International Journal of the Addictions*, 1968, *3*, 231.

Reinforcing Stimulus Functions of Drugs: Interpretations. I

Peter B. Dews

Department of Psychiatry
Harvard Medical School
Boston, Massachusetts

The organization of this book, according to ways in which drugs can function as stimulus would have been unthought of 15 years ago. Now behavioral pharmacology is dealing with defined and objectively measurable variables; one can see, at last, an end to the times when pharmacologists, scientists in dealing with other types of drug effects, were content to quote Shakespeare, De Quincey, and Huxley when giving an account of the behavioral effects of drugs.

A psychologic bias is evident in the papers presented here in that drugs are considered as stimuli. A cogent case could be made by a pharmacologist for considering stimuli as drugs. The general procedures for sorting out the multiple effects of a drug should be valuable for sorting out the multiple effects of a stimulus—certainly better suited than classical psychophysical procedures. Corresponding to dose-effect curves would be stimulus intensity-effect curves, and to drug antagonisms would be schedule antagonisms of stimulus effects. It was through drug studies that the ubiquitous importance of schedules of reinforcement were confirmed and clarified (Dews, 1963; Kelleher and Morse, 1968). Why not a similar contribution to stimulus control?

I will take it as proved that drug injections can maintain the behavior that precedes them, i.e., that drugs can function as reinforcers. What does this mean in the context of current views about reinforcement? Recent studies have led to such radical changes in how we think about reinforcement that the whole field of reinforcement theory has changed about, so that, while the answers are still the same (they have to be, since they are experimental findings), the ways in which we look at them have greatly changed.

The reason that studies on self-administration of drugs seemed important, when they were started, is probably summarized fairly by an anonymous writer in a publication on the status of research in pharmacology published recently by the National Institutes of Health (1967):

> Researchers long have had the ability to create drug dependence in the laboratory animal. Animals thus conditioned have provided science much valuable information as to the nature of the action of dependency-creating drugs, especially the hard narcotics. Unfortunately, however, the drug-dependent laboratory animal often raised more questions than he answered. The reason was inherent in the experimental procedure itself. The scientist could easily cause drug dependency in the laboratory animal. He could readily observe and quantitatively measure the physical and behavioral responses of the animal. But one essential factor was missing.
>
> That factor was free will—lacking in the animal because he, the drug-dependent animal, had to rely on the investigator for the maintenance of the drug habit. The investigator, in turn could only assess the animal's physical, not his psychological need for drugs. Free will, which plays a starring role in human drug dependency, thus was not contained in the experimental model.
>
> This major deficit in the study of drug dependency has now been largely overcome. Laboratory procedures have been developed which do provide free will to the drug-dependent animal. The drugs are available to the animal upon demand and enter his body directly, with no second party intervention, when the animal performs a simple, previously learned maneuver. The animal can thereby maintain his personal drug habit in accordance with his own desires as well as satisfy any physical need he feels for the drug at any given time. And since the investigator can control the total life situation of these "free-will" animal drug-dependents, and introduce pleasant as well as stressful experiences at will, greatly enlarged understanding of human drug dependency is soon forthcoming.

Psychologic theories—all of them, to the best of my knowledge—and common sense have agreed that reinforcers were either positive, with resulting behavior of seeking or maximizing, or negative, with resulting behavior of escaping from or minimizing. For example, electric shock at levels above a milliampere or so has been widely used as a noxious, aversive stimulus. Such shock can, in itself, serve no useful biologic purpose, and has been considered the pure negative reinforcer par excellence. Electric shock has proved highly effective in maintaining behavior which either terminates, or reduces the frequency or intensity of shock.

Electric shock can, however, also maintain behavior that *increases* the frequency of occurrence of shock. When squirrel monkeys wearing a collar and chain were subjected to an electric shock, they tended to pull on the chain. The chain was then attached to a switch and pulling on the chain was made to *deliver* shock to the monkey, according to a schedule. Under these circumstances responding (pulling the chain) was maintained, and the pattern of responding was appropriate to the schedule of shock delivery (Morse, Mead and Kelleher, 1967). Again, animals (monkeys and cats) have been trained under a schedule in which responses postpone shocks and have then been subjected, while responding, to the additional feature that every 10 or 15 minutes a response *delivers* a shock. When the schedule of shock postponement was subsequently removed, the animals responded with a fixed-interval pattern of responding, though the only consequence of the responding was the periodic delivery of electric shock (Byrd, 1969; McKearney, 1969). Finally, monkeys have been trained to work for food, self-administered shock superimposed, and then the food schedule discontinued, again with maintenance of responding solely by the self-administered shock (Kelleher and Morse, 1968).

There is, therefore, no doubt that self-administered shock can maintain responding. Now, of course, animals have to be *trained* to shock themselves. That the requirement of training is not, however, peculiar to shock-maintained responding is illustrated by a true anecdote. A number of years ago, Professor B.F. Skinner had a friend who was working in Philadelphia. The friend wrote that he would like to demonstrate pigeons pecking a key for food. He begged the loan of the appropriate demonstration apparatus. Professor Skinner obligingly shipped down to Philadelphia the apparatus and a couple of pigeons. The subsequent report was that the demonstration had been only half successful. One of the pigeons had refused to peck or perform at all appropriately in the demonstration. Inquiry elicited the following story. One of the pigeons had died, and had been replaced by a good Philadelphia pigeon. This was the one that, introduced unceremoniously and for the first time into the apparatus for the demonstration, had failed to perform. As a matter of fact, pigeons have to be trained to peck a key under a schedule of food presentation. Animals have also to be trained to work under a schedule of drug injection.

It is now clear that a wide variety of stimuli, including electric shocks and drugs, can function in a reinforcing mode, maintaining behavior on whose occurrence they are consequent. It is the rule rather than the exception that a stimulus can function as a reinforcer although every stimulus has its own characteristics as to how strongly and in what circumstances it will function as a reinforcer. For example, food functions well as a reinforcer when every response is followed by food, whereas shock has not maintained responding under this schedule (Kelleher and Morse, 1968). Among the relevant variables, the schedule is preeminent. To bring desires and free will into the picture merely obscures the real functional relationships. Let me repeat part of the quotation from the NIH publication, replacing "drug" by "shock."

> Laboratory procedures have been developed which do provide free will to the shock-dependent animal. The shocks are available to the animal upon demand, and enter his body directly, with no second party intervention, when the animal performs a simple, previously learned maneuver. The animal can thereby maintain his personal shock habit in accordance with his own desires as well as satisfy any physical need he feels for the shock at any given time.

The substitution is permissible since the evidence for "shock-dependency" is identical to the evidence for "drug-dependency" in subjects. The manifest absurdity of the transformed quotation illustrates the dangers of using a culturally derived view of the determinants of behavior to "explain" experimental findings, that is, of the dangers of prejudice in science. The dependence of the reinforcing effect of a stimulus on training and schedule is by no means confined to the examples mentioned; it is a general phenomenon. It will have to suffice here, however, to cite briefly another example recently published (Steiner, Beer and Shaffer, 1969). An electrode was implanted in the brain of an animal at a site such that the animal would press a lever to deliver electrical stimuli through the electrode. The exact temporal sequence of lever presses and consequent brain stimulations was recorded. When the same brain stimuli were delivered again to the animal in exactly the same temporal sequence, the animal would press a lever to turn off the stimuli, those same stimuli that had previously maintained lever pressing. This example of a stimulus changing its polarity from a positive mode to a negative mode complements the conversion from a negative mode to a positive mode of the strong electric shock in the experiments cited earlier.

Obviously, when drugs are studied as reinforcing stimuli, the stimulus control must be considered in terms of the history of the individual subject, the operating schedules and the parametric values of the stimuli (e.g., dose of drug), just as when other reinforcing stimuli are studied. This symposium has pioneered in bringing together information resulting from just such an approach.

Let us turn now to the problem of drug abuse. When I lectured to medical students on pharmacology 15 or so years ago, I used to hazard the guess that any drug that caused a reasonably prompt and significant behavioral effect would be liable to abuse. Morphine, alcohol and amphetamine all produce significant behavioral effects; they are grossly different drugs in almost all other respects, yet all are abused. The only property marihuana,

LSD, mescaline, chloroform, solvents of adhesives, nicotine, and so on seem to have in common is that they have significant behavioral effects and that they are abused by people. Perhaps correspondingly, Pickens and Thompson (Chapter 11) gave us a long list of drugs that have been shown to maintain self-administration behavior in animals. There does, however, seem to be an exception to the general rule, a drug, or rather a class of drugs, which has very significant and reasonably prompt behavioral effects, which has been widely available for almost 15 years, but which seems to be little abused, namely, phenothiazines related to chlorpromazine. The exception is the more remarkable because in the great majority of objective behavioral studies in mammals, chlorpromazine has effects that are very similar to, or indistinguishable from, morphine, which is the archetype of drugs of abuse. I recognize that pharmacologists in drug houses have been able to devise tests that distinguish between chlorpromazine and morphine, but these exceptions merely prove the rule; the tests that distinguish have been selected out of the great many that have been continued mainly *because* of their ability to identify morphine. In almost all ordinary objective behavioral testing situations, in reasonable doses, the similarities between chlorpromazine and morphine are much closer than between either of the drugs and members of any other class of drugs such as barbiturates, meprobamate, chlordiazepoxide, scopolamine, amphetamines, tetrahydrocannabinol and so on. Morphine certainly sustains self-administration behavior. Chlorpromazine is said not to, though this does not seem to be well documented in the literature. It would certainly seem worthwhile making a systematic comparison of the two drugs to see whether any particular behavioral attribute can be identified as related to the addictive potency of morphine and the lack of it of chlorpromazine. The studies might yield a clue as to the nature of the "antipsychotic" effects of phenothiazines.

REFERENCES

Byrd, L.D. Responding in the cat maintained under response-independent electric shock and response-produced electric shock. *J. Exp. Anal. Behav.*, 1969, *12*, 1-10.

Dews, P.B. *Schedules of Reinforcement*. Ciba Foundation Symposium, H. Steinberg, A.V.S. de Reuck and J. Knight, eds. London, J. & A. Churchill Ltd., 1964, 191-201.

Kelleher, R.T., and Morse, W.H. Determinants of the specificity of behavioral effects of drugs. *Ergebn. der Physiol.*, 1968, *60*, 1-56.

Kelleher, R.T., and Morse, W.H. Schedules using noxious stimuli. III. Responding maintained with response-produced electric shocks. *J. Exp. Anal. Behav.*, 1968, *11*, 819-838.

McKearney, J.W. Fixed-interval schedules of electric shock presentation: Extinction and recovery of performance under different shock intensities and fixed-interval durations. *J. Exp. Anal. Behav.*, 1969, *12*, 301-313.

Morse, W.H., Mead, R.N., and Kelleher, R.T. Modulation of elicited behavior by a fixed-interval schedule of electric shock presentation. *Science*, 1967, *157*, 215-217.

National Institutes of Health: Status of Research in Pharmacology and Toxicology: A Report by the Pharmacology and Toxicology Training Committee of the National Institute of General Medical Sciences, Bethesda, Md., 1967, 109-110.

Steiner, S.S., Beer, B., and Shaffer, M.M. Escape from self-produced rates of brain stimulation. *Science*, 1969, *163*, 90-91.

Reinforcing Stimulus Functions of Drugs: Interpretations. II

Kenneth MacCorquodale

Department of Psychology
University of Minnesota
Minneapolis, Minnesota

From the vantage point of the uninvolved but well-disposed observer the amount of information we are getting concerned the behavioral and stimulus properties of a wide variety of specific drugs is very impressive.

From the more general point of view, what has impressed me perhaps the most is the high degree of orderliness of these data. It seems to me that they contain few surprises in that the results are very congruent with what we know about the major dynamics of behavioral control. For example, once it is established that a drug is a discriminative stimulus, the discriminative behavior it controls is perfectly familiar and orderly; you would know it anywhere. It has its own parameter values of course but that is also predictable. If a drug is a reinforcer, it seems to sustain behavior in much the same way that any reinforcer does; if it is presented according to an intermittent schedule, the resultant behavior shows predictable scheduling effects. Many drugs appear to have discriminative, eliciting, and reinforcing properties, all three. But, as Professor Trapold suggested in his comments (Chapter 5), these properties do tend to go together, however mediately.

This consistency with other, more generally available, data may not seem very exciting to you, but a person working outside some new, active, and fast-moving area sometimes develops an anxiety that 'those others' know something that is about to pull the rug out from under him. I suppose this feeling explains in part why I accepted the invitation to be a discussant of these chapters. I did not dare not to.

But these studies are much more than merely consistent with our general views of the dynamics of behavior. They uniquely extend out knowledge of the molar processes involved. There are important questions which drug research can answer and which less "physiologic" research gives us relatively little clue to, such as the possibility of conditioning respondents by means of operant reinforcement, or the necessary and sufficient sites of action of stimulus application needed to achieve Pavlovian conditioning. These are important considerations because they show that this sector of research is not only illuminating with respect to the several properties of drugs as an object of principal interest, but they are also important avenues to information about the general and familiar processes of behavior.

Considering particularly the chapters concerned with the reinforcing properties of drugs, it is apparent that many drugs are reinforcers, and will be effective at dosages below those necessary to produce physical dependence. That, I think, was not very predictable. But, like all reinforcers, aside from their reinforcing effects they have little else in common in the way of behavioral side effects. That is the way it always seems to be with reinforcers, though. If it were not—if reinforcers had some consistent and unique side effects—we would be able to identify and define them independently of the behavior-strengthening effects, and thus get free of that restriction to postdiction of reinforcers that annoys the theorists and undergraduates so much.

One possibility that interested me particularly about drugs as reinforcers or, for that matter, as S^Ds, was that when they are presented, antithetic behavioral effects may very often, and perhaps most often, be expected. Drugs as drugs tend to disorganize behavior in diverse ways, or at least alter it. As reinforcers, and especially so if they are presented on some sort of intermittent schedule, they tend to organize it. Perhaps some of the anomalous effects of drug-reinforcement, especially priming, binges and self-regulated abstinence periods, are the products of cyclic processes during which behavior alternatively shows relatively more of one process and less of the other. Pickens and Thompson (Chapter 11) do, in fact, raise this possibility but they do not pursue it with any enthusiasm, although I take it that Woods and Schuster (Chapter 10) might. Probably Pickens and Thompson have some experimental evidence up their sleeves, which I am ignorant of, but I gather that in some part their mistrust of this possibility is due to the fact that during binges, and also following a priming injection, increases rather than decreases in response rates occur, suggesting that these drugs enhance rather than disrupt the reinforcement effect. However, I should think that an increased response rate can itself be a symptom of disruption, whose effects are simply additive with respect to the reinforcement effect and should therefore be separately accounted for.

I will predict, in any case, that whatever anomalies persist when drugs are used as reinforcers (such as priming, past experience, if these are indeed anomalous for reinforcers which I rather doubt) their biggest systematic or formal repercussions will be on our traditional notions concerning motivation rather than reinforcement as such. That is all right. Motivation is always in systematic and definitional trouble, it always has been and it apparently always will be. It is the first thing to wobble when a new reinforcer is discovered and analyzed, so drugs are in the best possible company in this respect.

I have said that these results seem most remarkable to me for their congruence with the effects of other stimulus manipulations. Let me hasten to say that this general orderliness and consistency pleases me, because it reassures me about the sensitivity and generality of our laboratory procedures, and the validity of the generalizations we have made so far about behavior in general. I suppose, however, that research workers in any specialized area would really prefer to get very durable, highly reproducible but wholly innovative and hopefully disconfirming outcomes. When this happens, one can get lots of extra mileage out of his results by brandishing a new paradigm at everyone else, or at least hinting at one, and proclaiming a scientific revolution. I have heard nothing of that sort here. We are all still in business so far as I can see, but we have a lot of new information about a new class of discriminative, eliciting, and reinforcing stimuli. That is news; it is useful and it is constructive. But it is not revolutionary, and I am delighted.

Index

Activity
  conditioning with drugs, 39-50
  unconditioned effects of drugs, 48
Apparatus
  habituation, 43
  influences on drug conditioning, 39-42

Behavioral history, 193-194

Central nervous system
  effective drugs, 89-92
  involvement in conditioning, 25-28
Concurrent reinforcement contingencies, 203-204
Conditioned drug effects
  Abstinence syndrome
    extinction, 62-63
    extinction in post-dependent monkeys, 63-66
    food reinforced behavior, 57-61
    morphine self-administration, 53-57
    reconditioning, 66-68
    sensitivity to nalorphine, 68-70
    situational conditioning, 61-62

Conditioned drug effects (cont.)
  Activity
    apparatus type, 39-42
    classical or operant conditioning, 49-50
    control group, 42
    factors influencing, 44-46
    habituation, 43
    new investigations, 46-49
  Cardiovascular
    bulbocapnine, 17-18
    conditional changes, 21-23
    conditioning with other stimuli, 28-32
    controls, 20-21
    drug effects on, 32-35
    involvement of CNS, 24-28
    modification of cardiovascular system, 16-17
    procedures, 18-20
Conditioned drug reinforcement, 205
Controls
  in drug reinforcement, 184-185
  of external stimuli, 142-146
  suitable groups, 42

Discrimination reversal, 128-130

219

Index

Discriminative stimulus function of drugs
  in free operant apparatus
    controls, 142-146
    discrimination reversal, 128-130
    drug probes, 130-131
    generalization, 125-128
    implications, 123-125
    procedure, 112, 134-135
    schedules
      food reinforcement, 113-122
      shock avoidance, 122-123
  in T-maze apparatus
    drugs and stimuli similarities, 94-97
    effective CNS drugs, 89-92
    peripherally acting drugs, 97-99
    procedures, 88-89
    relative effectiveness, 99-105
    various tasks, 92-94
Drug probes, 130-131
Drugs
  chronic effects, 182-184
  experience, 194-195
  peripherally acting, 97-99
  rate reducing effects, 169-172
  relative effectiveness, 99-105

Environmental stress, 197-198
Environmental variables influencing drug reinforcement
  current conditions, 197-204
    concurrent reinforcement contingencies, 203-204
    generalization, 198
    social, 198-203
    stress, 197-198
  motivational conditions, 195-197
    opiate dependence, 195-196
    stimulant dependence, 196-197
  prior history, 193-195
    behavioral history, 193-194
    drug experience, 194-195
  reinforcement variables, 205

Environmental variables influencing drug reinforcement (*cont.*)
    conditioned reinforcement, 205
    feedback, 205
Extinction
  in post-dependent monkeys, 63-66
  of conditioned activity, 45
  of nalorphine response, 62-63

Feedback stimuli, 205

Generalization, 125-128

Habituation, 43

Interoceptive stimulus control
  of behavior, 3-11
  discriminative control, 6-7
  in operant conditioning, 42-50
  in respondent conditioning, 3-6
  reinforcement control, 7-8
Interoceptors, 3
Interpretations
  discriminative stimulus functions, 149-150
  reinforcing stimulus functions, 209-217
  unconditioned stimulus functions, 73-83
Introduction, 3-11

Motivational conditions, 195-197

Operant conditioning
  classical or operant, 49-50
  interoceptive control by drugs, 6-7
  reinforcement by drugs, 7-8
Opiates as reinforcers
  effects of naloxone, 172-174

Opiates as reinforcers *(cont.)*
  low morphine doses, 165-169
  physical dependence, 164-165
  with prior drug treatment, 165
  rate reducing effects, 169-172

Past history, 193-195
Physical dependence, 164-165

Reconditioning abstinence syndrome, 66-68
Reinforcement schedules
  food, 113-122
  shock avoidance, 122-123
Reinforcement variables, 205
Reinforcing stimulus functions of drugs
  environmental variables, 193-208
  interpretations, 209-217
  opiates, 163-176
  stimulants, 177-192
Respondent conditioning
  classical or operant, 49-50
  of drug effects, 3-6
  procedure, 3-4

Situational conditioning, 61-62

Social influences, 198-203
Stimulants as reinforcers
  cautionary note, 190
  characteristics, 180-182
  chronic effects, 182-184
  controls, 184-185
  drugs, 177-178
  in rats, 180
  inhalation route, 186
  intravenous route, 186
  other animals, 185-186
  reinforcing doses, 178-179
  self-administration methods, 179-180
  variables, 186-190

Unconditioned stimulus function of drugs
  cardiovascular conditioning, 15-38
  interpretations, 73-83
  locomotor activity, 39-50
  on morphine self-administration, 51
  (See also conditioned abstinence, activity, and cardiovascular effects

Variables
  in activity conditioning, 44-46
  in stimulant reinforcement, 186-190

DATE DUE

DEC 1 1 1992

DEC 0 7 1995

DEMCO, INC. 38-2931